The
Brain Diet

The
Brain Diet

THE CONNECTION BETWEEN NUTRITION, MENTAL HEALTH, AND INTELLIGENCE

Alan C. Logan, ND, FRSH

Foreword by Martin Katzman, MD

CUMBERLAND HOUSE
NASHVILLE, TENNESSEE

THE BRAIN DIET

PUBLISHED BY CUMBERLAND HOUSE PUBLISHING
431 Harding Industrial Drive
Nashville, Tennessee 37211

Cover design: Gore Studio, Inc.

Library of Congress Cataloging-in-Publication Data

Logan, Alan C., 1967–
    The brain diet : the connection between nutrition, mental health, and intelligence /
Alan C. Logan ; foreword by Martin Katzman.
        p. cm.
    ISBN-13: 978-1-58182-508-4 (hardcover : alk. paper)
    ISBN-10: 1-58182-508-0 (hardcover : alk. paper)
    1. Brain. 2. Nutrition. 3. Mental health—Nutritional aspects. 4. Intellect—
Nutritional aspects. I. Title.
QP376.L64 2006
612.8'2—dc22
                                                                        2006004429

Printed in Canada
1 2 3 4 5 6 7—12 11 10 09 08 07 06

This book is dedicated to the brave souls who have struggled with a broken brain, and to the committed scientists, professionals, family, and friends who have worked tirelessly to help them.

With special thanks to all the kind tomodachies who welcomed and fed me such delicious brain food on my numerous trips to Japan . . . and to Yoshiko Sato, without whom this book would not have happened, I say, Sensei, domo arigato gozaimashita.

Thanks also to Dr. Martin Katzman and Dr. Alison Bested for the mentoring, Dr. Venket Rao for your open door, Dr. Tracey Beaulne for listening to me for hours on end, Dr. Andy Morgan III for showing me that it is never too late to take a new direction, and to Peg Baim and the members of Harvard's Mind-Body Medical Institute for having the confidence to allow me to take the podium.

To my parents and family, thanks for always standing by me.

CONTENTS

Foreword

Nutritional neuroscience is one of the hottest areas of current scientific investigation, yet sadly, it is an area with which most clinical mental health professionals are unfamiliar. Nutrition has historically been glossed over in medical schools and in most postgraduate mental health programs. Fortunately, this dismissal of nutrition and its relation to mental health is slowly changing.

Scientific studies over the last decade or so have shown strong links between nutrition and both neurological and psychiatric conditions. The food choices made during pregnancy, lactation, and early childhood may have long term consequences on child development, intelligence, and behavior. Furthermore, as our waistlines expand in North America, it appears that we are setting the stage for a later reduction in brain power, or even a literal shrinking of the brain, according to some new research. The same foods that promote weight gain are the same foods that can compromise brain function by promoting inflammation and free radical generation. Research shows that stress, in addition to being directly damaging to delicate nerve cells, can drive inappropriate food choices, further interfere with brain function, and promote weight gain. As such, choosing the right foods and eating in the right state of mind can ensure that we perform at our brain's maximum ability.

I have known Alan Logan for the past six years, ever since he helped out on a research project of mine while in naturopathic medical school. Since then he has grown to become one of North America's leading experts on nutritional medicine. Alan's original theories and ideas have been published in many mainstream medical journals, and his recent article concerning omega-3 fatty acids and depression has become the most accessed article since the inception of the journal *Lipids in Health and Disease*. We have published research together and have a number of exciting projects in the pipeline. In a just a short time, Alan has gone from taking courses at Harvard Medical School's Mind-Body Medical Institute to being part of the faculty in Harvard's continuing medical education program. Many hold themselves out to be "experts" in nutrition and dietary supplements these days, but when Harvard's Mind-Body Medical Institute needed an authority for lectures on the topic, they knocked on Dr. Logan's door.

I knew when I first met Alan that he was a progressive thinker, well capable of synthesizing complex science into clear and clinically useful ideas. It is not at all surprising to me that Alan would be the first author to translate countless scientific studies from various disciplines into a reader-friendly guide to brain health. This is by far the most thorough and comprehensive text written on the topic of nutrition and brain health, one that should capture the attention of both medical professionals and the general populace.

With its practical advice, *The Brain Diet* is sure to make a significant difference in the lives of many individuals. However, it is also a shout out to greater society . . . a wake-up call that must be answered. Alan's examination of the rapid Westernization of the Japanese diet, which appears to run hand in hand with increases in depression, behavioral problems, school violence, and crime, is an eye-opening discussion with enormous implications for all of us.

The brain is completely reliant upon quality nutrition for both its structure and its function—no matter how far we advance technologically, this is a constant that will never change. If you want to maximize your potential in life, you must support your brain nutritionally. While nutritional medicine appears to play a role in the prevention and treatment of certain brain-related conditions, I appreciate Alan's conservative approach when it comes to proper interventions. As pointed out numerous times in this book, brain conditions, both neurological and psychiatric, can be very serious—nutrition and certain supplements are never a substitute for appropriate medical care. The principles of *The Brain Diet* plan can be incorporated into the treatment of most brain conditions as a supervised adjunctive measure.

The Brain Diet is ultimately a book about the promotion of health, not just of the brain, but of the entire body. In many ways it is ahead of its time—in the coming years, nutritional neuroscience is destined to become part of the training of all professions that are involved with conditions of the human brain. If you want to maximize your potential in life, you must support your brain nutritionally. *The Brain Diet* will be a classic at the forefront of a new era of brain science.

Yours in health,
Martin Katzman, MD, FRCP(C)
Assistant Professor, Psychiatry
University of Toronto
Medical Director, START Clinic for
Mood and Anxiety Disorders
790 Bay Street Suite 900
Toronto, Ontario M5G 1N8

Introduction

The idea that our dietary choices can influence health is certainly not a new one. Most people are well aware that nutrition can play a role in various medical conditions, most notably cardiovascular disease and cancer. But what about depression, anxiety, multiple sclerosis, Parkinson's disease, Alzheimer's disease, migraine headaches, attention deficit hyperactivity disorder, and other neurological and psychiatric conditions? Is it possible that nutritional choices might influence these disorders, and is it possible that diet might make a difference in overall mood and well-being as well? Modern scientific research, as outlined in the pages of this book, demonstrates that not only can nutrition influence mood and well-being over the short term, there is emerging evidence that dietary choices are playing an entirely undervalued role in the prevention and treatment of neurological and psychiatric (neuropsychiatric) conditions.

Food is in abundance in developed counties—it is not difficult to find a quick and easy calorie fix when we need one—but what are we eating? The answer is largely foods that are devoid of fiber, vitamins, minerals, antioxidants, and the critically important omega-3 fatty acids. Nutritional intake for many North Americas is subpar. Startling research in the journal *Food Review* (2002) shows that only five foods—canned tomatoes, fresh and frozen potatoes, iceberg lettuce, and onions—account for 50 percent of our total vegetable consumption. This is not a joke; we're talking about the trimmings on a hamburger and a side of fries. Despite the availability of fruits and vegetables in the produce section of supermarkets, there is a clear lack of variety in the diets of most North Americans. Fruits and vegetables are our greatest source of phytonutrients, naturally occurring antioxidants within the colored pigments and fiber of plants. Phytonutrients have been referred to in scientific journals as guardians of our health, and the latest research suggests that this also includes mental and neurological health. The rates of mental and neurological disorders are rapidly on the rise, and aside from environmental and nutritional influence, scientists offer little in the way of explanations. Genetic influences can explain neurological and psychiatric conditions to some degree, but even in identical twins—who share the same genetics—it appears that genes are responsible for 50 percent or fewer of most brain conditions. Environment is also a huge factor. Daily stressors, social networks, beliefs, humor, optimism, history of trauma, and levels of physical activity are among many factors that can influence the development and course of neurological and psychiatric conditions. You can now add nutrition to that list.

We all come into this world with genetic susceptibilities, some for neurological conditions, some for diabetes, cancer, etc.; researchers are now finding that nutrition can influence genetic expression; in other words, whether or not, or to what degree, a susceptible individual will actually go on to have a certain condition may be influenced by nutrition. This area of study is known as nutritional genomics, and it is certainly the future of medicine.

Antioxidant phytonutrients found in nature, and on a minority of dinner plates (those who take five or more daily servings of fruits and vegetables), appear to be key players in the nutritional genomics revolution. As mentioned, most North Americans are well aware of the connections between nutrition and heart health or diabetes. The jump from the well-known benefits of nutrition on cardiovascular health (for example) to mental health is not really a leap at all, it is a small and simple step. Consider that all of the nutrients that are heart healthy, omega-3 fatty acids from fish and seafood, fiber-rich whole grains, dark green and other colorful vegetables, nuts, various vitamins, minerals, and antioxidants are not just for the heart. Research is showing that these same dietary items are equally important in the promotion of brain health.

Consider also that your brain is 60 percent fat and is reflective, in its fat makeup, of your personal dietary fat intake. Today we are overconsuming saturated fats, trans fats and omega-6 rich oils, such as corn and safflower; these dietary changes may be changing brain chemistry—and not for the better. The delicate brain cells require the same antioxidant support that the heart and blood vessels need to preserve structure and function. Important dietary B vitamins such as folic acid, vitamin B12 and vitamin B6 can lower the risk of cardiovascular disease, and interestingly, exciting new research shows that they can also help with depression. Consider that if a person has just one episode of major depression in a lifetime, he or she is almost three times more likely to die of cardiovascular disease later on.

It is sad that only a relatively small group of international researchers have devoted themselves to investigating the link between nutrition and the brain. The good news is that their high-quality and groundbreaking research, which I have compiled and will share with you in this book, has opened the eyes of many other scientists—and it's not a moment too soon. We have a mental health crisis on our hands right now. According to the largest national survey of its kind, published in the *Archives of General Psychiatry* (2005), all mental health conditions are on the rise. Incredibly, one in every two Americans can expect to have a diagnosable mental health condition at some point in their life. More and more young adults are turning to sleep medications and more than 1.5 million North American adults are now on medications for attention deficit and hyperactivity. Neurological conditions are also on the rise. Real people are suffering in the here and now with emotional and neurological conditions, and many more are on an unseen road to illness . . . education and public awareness of nutritional influences on brain health are desperately needed.

As I hope you will see, as a scientist, I am very passionate about this topic. I remain fascinated by the phrase "you are what you eat." I have lived with tremendous anxiety in my life and am also well aware, from a personal perspective, of the nutritional influences on mood. However, this book is not about my personal anecdotal experiences, it is about credible, published science.

It is also important to understand that nutritional changes, dietary supplements, and herbal remedies are not a substitute for appropriate medical treatment. Those with diagnosed mental and neurological conditions, or those with related symptoms, should be guided by a mental health professional or neurologist depending on the illness. However, many mental health care providers and neurologists may be pleasantly surprised by the outcomes when brain-friendly nutrition is incorporated into their treatment approach.

To quote Dr. David Horrobin (1939–2003) from the journal *International Psychogeriatrics*, "Trying to apply any treatment modality, whether psychological, pharmacological, or social, to a brain that cannot function normally because of lack of an essential nutrient is like trying to run a 220-volt electrical appliance on a 120-volt system." Dr. Horrobin, an Oxford University medical graduate, will always be remembered as the founding father of the specialty area that examines nutritional influences on the health of the brain. His thirty years of research on essential fatty acids and other nutritional factors finally brought the role of diet in behavior and cognition to a respected level. Thankfully, Dr. Horrobin was able to see the fruits of his labor before he passed away; in a flurry of impressive studies published in prestigious medical journals, he showed that omega-3 fatty acids can improve many of the symptoms of depression, schizophrenia, and other brain-related conditions. Dr. Horrobin's original work continues to drive research in the area now called nutritional neuroscience.

I sincerely hope that you will find the research and ideas in the following chapters helpful, and that you will share it with others. Of course, brain nutrition is most suited to prevention, so that is where the emphasis should be. Let's get the message out . . . proper nutrition, physical activity, and lifestyle habits are not only good for the heart, they are also good for the brain.

Yours in health,
Dr. Alan C. Logan
Naturopathic Physician

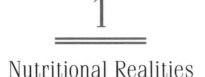

1

Nutritional Realities

T HE BRAIN HAS BEEN DESCRIBED as the final frontier in medicine—with 100 billion nerve cells (neurons) and even greater numbers of supporting cells (neuroglia) it is unquestionably our most complex organ. The brain is the conductor of the body's orchestra; it directs our thoughts, actions, emotions, and basic desires. It is responsible for regulating activities that we hardly ever think about—such as heartbeat and respiratory rates, wakefulness and sleep, and digestive functions, to name a few. Given the immense workload of the brain, it shouldn't be too surprising that it takes up and utilizes 20 percent of the entire energy supply of the body. Where does this energy supply come from? The answer is simple—your diet. Not only does the diet supply fuel to support proper functioning of the brain, it also supports the structure, or the scaffolding of the brain. What you put into your mouth has both short- and long-term consequences on brain functioning and structure. As you will see, a variety of important nutrients (vitamins, minerals, carbohydrates, proteins, fats, and plant-based phytonutrients) are critical for the performance and long-term maintenance of the brain.

As scientists begin to uncover the intricate anatomy and physiology of the brain, it is becoming clear that we have historically underestimated nutritional influences on mental and neurological health. This area of research, termed *nutritional neuroscience*, is barely in its infancy, yet tremendous discoveries have already been made. The sad nutritional realities of the modern diet are not supportive of optimal functioning and survival of the brain. Yes, we can get by on low-quality nutrition and fast food, but it definitely takes away our mental edge and clogs up the brain over time. Scientific research is showing us that the brain demands "premium" dietary fuel, yet most North Americans are running their brain on "regular" fuel. Inadequate brain nutrition sets the stage for inadequate brain performance, and less protection against the daily grind and wear and tear of life. Before examining the dietary interventions that may be helpful in various neurological and psychiatric conditions, let's first look at the nutritional realities as they exist in North America. Where do North Americans get their nutritional fuel from, and what voids exist in today's diet? These are important questions with significant brain consequences.

Macronutrients

The dietary macronutrients are the main nutritional players; they are carbohydrates, proteins, and fats. For the last thirty years we have seen one fad after another with regard to which macronutrient is best and which group should be restricted. In the late '70s and '80s we had the fat-free fiasco and at the dawn of the new century we had the no-carb craze. While this nutritional nonsense generated huge profits for the food companies and restaurants that propagated the myths, there was relatively little reward for the consumers, particularly in brain health. Consider that the brain itself is 60 percent fat and relies upon dietary fat to ensure proper structure and function. Consider that complex carbohydrates provide a steady stream of fuel for the brain and, without them, certain proteins (amino acids) that form important chemical messengers (neurotransmitters) in the brain will be less available.

I heard time and time again from those on the high-protein and carbohydrate-restricted diets that they were irritable and had low energy despite the fact that they were losing weight. A 2003 study from Dr. Brian Butki and colleagues at Southern Illinois University showed that those on an Atkins-based diet reported higher levels of fatigue and decreased mood, and did not have the normal feel-good response to physical activity. Take away complex carbohydrates and you take away the body's primary energy source.

In addition, complex carbohydrates, i.e. whole grains such as brown rice, whole wheat, and oat bran, provide essential nutrients critical to brain function. I am always leery when I see a dietary regimen (such as the low-carb) that recommends a daily multivitamin/mineral to make up for essential nutrients that may become deficient simply through adherence. As I will discuss shortly, the North American nutritional intake already has some gaping holes to begin with, so why add more?

Out of the ashes of nutritional fads has arisen two very important considerations: There are good fats and bad fats, and there are good carbs and bad carbs. Of course, it is the good in both categories that support acute and long-term brain health. Despite these lessons, some sad realities remain. Consider that the most significant source of carbohydrates, cereal grains, accounts for 24 percent of our total percentage energy intake. However, only a measly 3.5 percent of our energy from grains is accounted for by whole grains, a sad state indeed. The intake of refined sugars in Western countries has increased eightfold in the last two hundred years, and more recently the intake of high-fructose corn syrup—as found in soft drinks—has increased from 0.5 pounds per capita in 1970 to more than 60 pounds per capita in 1997! While these simple sugars provide a temporary boost, its like fool's gold for the brain. Within a very short period of time there will be a significant drop in blood sugar, and then the brain is gasping for more. Complex carbohydrates provide a slow and steady stream of energy and vital nutrients. Simple sugars are known as empty calories and, as far as the brain goes, they are an empty promise. Like the guy who never calls for a second date, simple sugars leave the neurons (nerve cells) waiting by the phone.

The quick sugar fix is associated with an increased risk of diabetes and cardiovascular disease by way of spiking blood sugar and increased insulin secretion. Insulin is responsible for guiding sugar into our blood cells for use and storage. Over time, the cells can become resistant to the constant bombardment of high insulin levels. Eventually it takes a lot more insulin to do the work of sugar guidance and in time this takes a huge toll. While cardiovascular disease and diabetes are well known to be associated with high insulin resistance, new research shows that elevated insulin (hyperinsulinemia) is also a risk factor for neurodegenerative diseases such as

Alzheimer's and psychiatric conditions such as depression. Indeed, per capita sugar consumption in various nations is associated with increased rates of depression and severe forms of mental illness. I will focus on these nutritional areas in more detail as the chapters unfold, but suffice to say that simple sugars provide only a brief energy fix, one that ultimately drags the brain down.

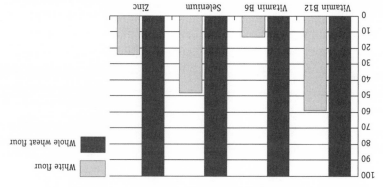

Levels of four important nutrients after the refining of whole wheat flour. Low levels of each of these nutrients have been associated with human depression.

While scientists are mapping out the complex mechanisms behind the negative consequences of sugar consumption and insulin resistance on brain health, at a fundamental level oxidative stress is a key player. Oxidative stress appears to be at least one mechanism by which high sugar and high insulin levels can damage cells. Indeed, high-fructose corn syrup from soda has been shown to increase oxidative stress and lower antioxidant blood levels for up to four hours after consumption of a single can. Oxidative stress, a consequence of normal day to day living and breathing, is normally kept in check by the elaborate antioxidant pathways in the body. We rely upon dietary nutrients to keep the antioxidant defense system in top working order. Free radical production (oxidative stress) can damage delicate brain cells. As you will see, increased oxidative stress is a common thread among various neurological and emotional disorders.

Fats have had a bad reputation for years; the fat-free craze and vilification of fats was like arresting an entire community in an effort to catch a few criminals. In terms of fat, the real "criminals" are saturated and man-altered fats called trans fatty acids. These two bad guys are now known to be associated with a variety of medical conditions and subpar brain health. Saturated and trans fats are solid fats, hard at room temperature. When you look at a piece of meat in a supermarket and see the white marble, you are looking at saturated fat. Butter, fatty meets, cheese, margarine, milk, and baked goods are all sources of saturated fat. Trans fats used to be liquid fats before they were transformed into hard fats for use in margarines and a host of baked goods. Trans fats are "fake fats" that will be listed as "hydrogenated vegetable oil" or "shortening." New government regulations ensure that consumers can identify the trans fat content on food labels.

Despite reductions in overall fat intake, we are still consuming 15 percent of our total energy as saturated fat, and more than 7 percent of our daily fatty acid intake is in the form of trans fats. This is a sad state when you consider that the Institute of Medicine reminds us that "saturated fats, trans fatty acids, and dietary cholesterol have no known beneficial role in preventing chronic disease and are not required at any level in the diet . . . the recommendation is to keep their intake as low as possible" (Institute of Medicine 2002, *Dietary Reference Intakes for Energy, Carbohydrate, Fiber, Fatty Acids, Cholesterol, Protein, Amino Acids*). Both of these fats have been shown to elevate the risk of cardiovascular disease. Research indicates that our bodies really don't know what to make of trans fats, and they wreak havoc, promoting inflammation, elevating cholesterol, and increasing the risk of diabetes. Gram-for-gram, trans fats increase the risk of cardiovascular blockage by more than tenfold versus saturated fats. When you can identify dietary agents such as saturated and trans fats that promote inflammation, disturb blood sugar levels, and compromise blood flow, you can be assured that they will have a negative impact on brain health.

There are two groups of fats that we absolutely do need—omega-3 and omega-6 fatty acids. These groups are known as essential because we cannot make them on our own, so we rely upon dietary intake. The essential fatty acids keep the brain fluid, or well-oiled. These essential fatty acids are part of the special coating around all nerve cells known as the neuronal membrane. The neuronal membrane is designed to be supple, flexible, or "fluid," as it must accommodate the passage of certain important messengers through tiny pores. If the neuronal membrane is fed a diet of saturated fats, cholesterol, and trans fats, it becomes hard and inflexible. The neuronal membrane is a good reflection of your dietary fat choices. In states of omega-3 and omega-6 fatty acid deficiency and over-consumption of saturated fats, the communication from nerve cell to nerve cell becomes compromised due to an inflexible membrane. For many individuals, dietary fat choices may influence the development and treatment outcomes of neurological and psychiatric conditions.

When it comes to optimal brain function, it is the omega-3 fatty acids that we really need to consider. Omega-6 fatty acids (as found in corn, safflower, sunflower, and soybean oils) are everywhere, and a deficiency is virtually an impossibility. In fact, in 1999 an international panel of thirty of the world's leading fat experts convened in Washington, D.C., and recommended that the dietary omega-6 to omega-3 intake ratio should be about 2:1. In North America today, omega-6 fats outnumber omega-3 by anywhere between 10:1 and 20:1. As important as omega-6 fatty acids are, a large number of studies have shown that they can promote inflammation, particularly when taken in excess. Omega-6 fatty acids might play a role in a number of neurological and psychiatric conditions.

Much like oxidative stress, inflammation, even at low levels, is a common thread among neurological and psychiatric conditions. Omega-3 fatty acids, on the other hand, have been shown to be anti-inflammatory in the body, and to be beneficial in a number of behavioral and neurological conditions. Sadly, North American intake of two key omega-3 fatty acids, docosahexaenoic acid (DHA), and eicosapentaenoic acid (EPA), is a paltry combined 130 mg per day. Consider that the aforementioned international panel of fat experts recommended a minimum of 650 mg of EPA/DHA per day. Clearly we have a nutritional void to fill when it comes to omega-3. Emerging research shows the importance of DHA for pregnancy, brain development, learning, and the prevention of cognitive decline later in life. EPA is critical in regulating mood, with clinical studies showing it is helpful in depression and in lowering inflammation. Indeed it is clear that these two omega-3 fatty acids, EPA and DHA, are vital for brain health from conception through old age.

Dietary protein provides critically important amino acids that are used in the manufacture of behavior and mood regulating brain chemicals known as neurotransmitters. For example, the amino acid tryptophan is found in milk and turkey, and this gets converted into the so-called "feel-good" neurotransmitter called serotonin. This conversion of tryptophan into serotonin requires certain vitamins and is optimized in the presence of carbohydrates. That's why so many people feel relaxed and sleepy when they finish eating Thanksgiving dinner. The tryptophan from the turkey gains access to the brain in the presence of sweet potato, stuffing, and cranberry sauce. The tryptophan and turkey connection is pretty well known, and any *Seinfeld* fan will remember the episode where Jerry "drugs" his girlfriend with turkey and wine to make her sleepy. Other amino acids are critical for the manufacture of mood and energy regulating dopamine and gamma amino butyric acid (GABA) neurotransmitters. Research suggests that foods and certain dietary supplements may be helpful in a variety of psychiatric and neurological conditions due to their ability to influence neurotransmitters. These will be discussed in more detail later; for now it is important to recognize the overall importance of dietary protein from lean meats, low-fat dairy, soy, eggs, and fish.

Whey protein, from dairy, is a great way to ensure adequate intake of high-quality protein without the added saturated fat. North Americans are generally not lacking in protein intake; it's the *context* of the dietary protein that leads to problems. Often, protein is consumed by way of processed meats, whole milk, cheese, and fatty cuts of beef. The much-needed amino acids are found in these protein sources, but over the long term the chemicals and saturated fats assault the brain. Consider too, that the nutritional makeup of animal tissue is reflective of its dietary intake of fatty acids, and today's animal rearing practices (grain feeding) have led to much higher levels of omega-6 fatty acids in the meat that you eat. Animals that are free-range and allowed to forage on green grasses have much higher levels of brain healthy omega-3 fatty acids. As pointed out by Michael Pollan in his brilliant exposé on animal rearing in the *New York Times Magazine* ("This Steer's Life," March 31, 2002), the old saying "you are what you eat" should be changed to "you are what *what you eat* eats"!! Thankfully, free-range meats, including buffalo, and free-range, high omega-3 eggs are becoming more readily available.

Micronutrients and Phytonutrients

Micronutrients are your vitamins and minerals; they are critical for optimal brain function but are sadly lacking in today's North American diet.

It is hard to believe, but even today with huge supermarkets filled with a vast variety of foods, we are still deficient in so many vitamins and minerals. Despite cereal fortification, 33 percent of Americans are not meeting the minimum recommendations for folic acid. Consider that at least half of the U.S. population does not meet the recommended dietary allowance (RDA) for important brain vitamins and minerals, including calcium, magnesium, zinc, vitamin A, and vitamin B6. These are the minimal recommended intakes! Low dietary zinc in particular is worrisome because zinc has an important role in brain function. Recent studies have shown that low levels of zinc are associated with fatigue, depression, and poor mental performance. Yet in our society we tend to bypass the dietary solution of whole grains, nuts, and seafood, and instead reach for a sugar-laden commercial energy drink.

One of the main reasons for these micronutrient inadequacies is the reliance upon refined sugars, which are devoid of nutrients, as a primary energy source. When whole grains, seafood, fruits, and vegetables are replaced by processed foods, fatty meats, and liquid candy in the form of soft drinks and other simple carbohydrates, the obvious consequence is a loss of critical vitamins and minerals. As we will see in the following chapters, such micronutrient deficiencies are not without neurological and psychiatric consequences.

Plant foods are known to contain not only vitamins and minerals but also 25,000-plus microchemicals that give plants their color, taste, and texture. These so-called phytochemicals include plant pigments, which have potent antioxidant activities. The bulk of the research on phytochemicals shows they can help prevent cardiovascular disease and cancer; however, exciting new studies show that they are also extremely important in protecting the delicate cells of the nervous system. It is not surprising that phytochemicals are of such benefit in human health when you consider that they are manufactured in plants as a defense mechanism for the purpose of their *own* survival and health.

One of the largest and best known groups of phytochemicals is the polyphenol group. Within this family are the flavonoids, which include flavones, flavonols, flavanones, catechins, anthocyanins, and isoflavones. To provide a full spectrum of phytochemical protection, we need to consume a variety of fruits, vegetables, and plant-based beverages. Consider that the catechins are found in high amounts in green tea; the antho-

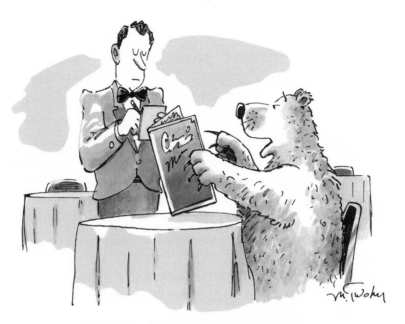

"I shouldn't, but I'm going to have the garbage."

cyanins in blueberries, cherries, and elderberry; the isoflavones in soy; flavonols in apples; and on and on. There are other important groups of phytochemicals, including the carotenoid family, which is made up of beta-carotene, lutein, lycopene, and zeaxanthin. Beta-carotene is found in carrots and other orange vegetables, lutein in dark greens such as broccoli and kale, lycopene in red vegetables such as red peppers and tomatoes, and zeaxanthin in yellow and green vegetables such as corn and spinach. In addition, there are other beneficial phytochemicals such as limonene in citrus fruits; ellagic acid in berries; and sulforaphane in Brussels sprouts, kale, cabbage, and broccoli. Again, North Americans have access to such a wide variety of fruits and vegetables, yet the research clearly shows that we are simply not taking advantage of the entire color spectrum of brain-protecting phytochemicals.

Despite the efforts of government and private nutrition education groups and volumes of international research supporting the benefits, the fact remains that North Americans are just not eating enough fruits and vegetables. Some research provides inflated figures when it comes to consumption of vegetables, but a closer look reveals sad nutritional realities. Four foods account for half of the total vegetable intake in adults—

potatoes (mostly frozen and fried), iceberg lettuce, onions, and tomatoes. As mentioned earlier, it is indeed the trimmings on a burger and a side of fries! Dark green and deep yellow vegetables combine to account for only 6 to 8 percent of vegetable intake. Even when potatoes and tomatoes are included, research shows that only 20 percent of adults eat three servings of vegetables and two serving of fruits per day. As of 2005, it is now recommended that we consume seven to nine servings of vegetables and fruits per day! On a given day, almost half of adults consume no fruit at all and, as with vegetables, variety is absent. Most fruit servings are consumed as orange juice, certainly a health beverage packed with vitamin C, but a greater variety is required to maximize your health. College students are notoriously low in fruit and vegetable intake; even when fried potato is included, they fall short in both categories. Of course, they comply with the meat (mostly high fat, processed) and grain (mostly processed, low-fiber) groups, passing them with flying colors.

What really upsets me are the statistics related to fruit and vegetable intake among children; the dietary intake of children will not only affect their delicate brains today, they may be habit-forming and influence lifetime brain function and longevity. Only 7 percent of children consume three or more servings of vegetables and two or more servings of fruit. As with adults, half of all children surveyed consumed less than one serving of fruit per day and fried potatoes account for the majority of the vegetable intake. When fried vegetables are excluded, 30 percent of children consume less than one vegetable serving per day. These are nutritional inadequacies with acute and long-term consequences.

Top Food Choices as Reported by 227 Public High School Foodservice Directors

pizza	fat-containing baked goods
hamburgers	fried potatoes
sandwiches	salty, fat-containing snacks
cookies	sweetened beverages
crackers	

(ADAPTED FROM PROBART, ET AL, JOURNAL OF THE AMERICAN DIETETIC ASSOCIATION, 2005)

Other Considerations

In addition to the nutritional voids of vitamins/minerals, omega-3 fatty acids, and phytochemicals, a fourth gaping hole is that of fiber intake. Fiber is the component of plants that the human body is unable to digest. Dietary fiber intake is subpar, and its absence may have implications way beyond the gastrointestinal tract. North Americans are consuming only 13 grams of fiber per day, at least one-third less than traditional diets consumed a century ago. We should be anywhere from 7 to 25 grams higher, depending on age and gender. Dietary fiber is the great detoxifier; it can help to eliminate toxins such as heavy metals and hormonal by-products that can disturb cognitive function. Fiber intake is well known to help maintain a lean body, lower oxidative stress, and reduce the risk of cardiovascular disease and type 2 diabetes. Again, dietary factors that can lower the risk of clogged arteries and blood sugar imbalances are turning out to be important in brain health. Beyond this, dietary fiber may influence the growth of certain bacteria in the gut—these are the so-called friendly bacteria, which provide numerous health benefits.

Daily Fiber Requirements	
AGE	DAILY FIBER* NEEDED
Men 14–50	38 g
Women 14–50	25 g
Men over 50	30 g
Women over 50	21 g
Children 2–13	5 g

*The recommended daily Adequate Intake (AI) of total fiber as per the U.S. National Academy of Sciences and Health Canada. The typical fiber intake for adults is currently 13 g.

Dr. Martin Katzman of the University of Toronto and I have gathered the scientific data from various medical disciplines to show that bacteria in the gut have the potential to influence mood and behavior. Dietary fiber has a profound effect on beneficial bacteria. In our article published in the journal *Medical Hypotheses* (2005), we provide ample evidence indicating that what is happening inside the gut may be influencing depression and other neuropsychiatric conditions. I will discuss this in more detail in the Gut-Brain chapter. Increasing fruits, vegetables, and whole grains in the daily diet will automatically increase total dietary fiber.

The Stage Is Set

Clearly, huge nutritional voids exist in North American nutrition, yet so many are apparently getting by just fine. You can probably think of many of your friends or co-workers who live on fast food, never let a green vegetable pass their lips, and enjoy an ample supply of ice cream, chips, and candy. They may seem healthy and immune from the colds and viruses that many "healthy" eaters seem to succumb to. A small minority of these individuals will defy the nutritional odds, living into old age and remaining fairly healthy. We all know one or two people like this, or the proverbial heavy smoker who lived until he was ninety. The vast majority of unhealthy eaters will, however, succumb to the nutritional influences on genetics, i.e. the influence of saturated fats and sugars (and the absence of protective vitamins, minerals, good fats, fiber, and phytochemicals) on the genetic expression of cardiovascular disease, cancer, diabetes, and a long list of neurodegenerative and psychiatric conditions. Thanks to the emerging research in the discipline known as "nutritional genomics" (or nutrigenomics), we now know that nutrition plays a role in whether or not, and to what degree, an illness may present itself. Consider diabetes (Type II), where healthy dietary modifications can reverse the illness in some individuals. In this case, the expression of genetic information is altered by changing one environmental variable. In diabetes, and in many of the neuropsychiatric cases to be discussed here, the environmental variable that can influence the disease onset and/or its course is nutrition. Consider that all humans are 99.9 percent identical in terms of gene sequence; the 0.1 percent variation in sequence accounts for differences in hair and skin color and other obvious differences, but most importantly, the susceptibility to disease. However, the hundreds of published studies involving identical twins have taught us that susceptibility to disease is only mediated in part by gene sequence. If genetics were the whole story, then identical twins (who share exactly the same gene sequence) would always have the same neurological and psychiatric conditions as

• • • CASE REPORT • • •

Todd is a forty-two-year-old retail manager who had been diagnosed with depression. He had a history of depressive symptoms that had waxed and waned for a number of years. His psychiatrist had tried different anti-depressant medications over the years with varying degrees of success. He reported that after a two-month trial, his latest antidepressant was not making much of difference and his mood was still low.

Todd was placed on a multivitamin/mineral formula to ensure adequate intake of folic acid, which has been shown in clinical research to enhance the effectiveness of antidepressant medications. The multivitamin/mineral formula also provided selenium and vitamin B12, which have been noted to be low in depression. In addition, Todd was placed on 300 micrograms of chromium picolinate, which has been shown to be helpful in new depression studies. Based on separate research, a high-EPA fish oil formula (o3mega+ joy™) was added to provide 1000 mg of EPA per day. Todd disclosed all three supplements to his treating psychiatrist.

In addition to the supplements, Todd made a concerted effort to change some dietary habits as well. Like many patients with depression, he had significant sugar cravings and a real desire for sweet foods and beverages. A review of his diet diary revealed little in the way of complex, whole-grain carbohydrates. The deep-colored fruits and vegetables that provide important antioxidant support in depression were alien foods in Todd's world, and fish intake was reported to be an occasional fried fast-food patty. Whole grains and oily fish were worked into his meal plans, and high-antioxidant fruits and vegetables became daily dietary items.

Within two weeks of being on this protocol, Todd reported significant improvements. Whether the diet and supplements were directly responsible, or whether they allowed the antidepressant to work more effectively, we don't know. It really doesn't matter much to Todd, who has since experienced major improvements in his quality of life.

they proceed through life. Of course that is not the case: Nutrition, stressors, social support, mental outlook, self-esteem, and a host of environmental factors can account for the fact that less than 50 percent of sets of identical twins share most neurological and psychiatric disorders.

When it comes to brain nutrition and enhancing daily mental performance, as well as putting the brakes on the development of neurological and behavioral-emotional disorders, you must first fill in the nutritional voids. The preservation of the brain is a lifelong nutritional effort, and there are enormous advantages when you stick with the Brain Diet. Gains include mental sharpness, an edge in a competitive world; improved mood; increased mental focus; prevention of brain-related diseases and ailments; decreased risk of cognitive decline; and an improved quality of life in the older years.

Let's have a closer look at oxidative stress. . . .

2

Cutting the Common Threads: Oxidative Stress and Inflammation

Oxidative Stress

Despite being relatively light in weight, at just 2 percent of total adult body weight, the human brain demands an enormous amount of energy and blood flow for optimal performance. Our ability to think, to reason, to create art and music, to develop technology, to perform complex tasks, and much, much more that we often take for granted is a consequence of brain activity. The electrochemical processes involved in brain activity generate free radicals, which take a toll in the form of oxidative stress. Free radicals are chemical "thugs," which steal electrons from other molecules. This process of armed robbery (loss of electrons) is called oxidation, and the free radical hoodlums are in a gang called "oxidizing agents," also known as reactive oxygen species. These gang members are more than capable of causing damage to delicate brain cells. However, the brain has a tight security operation known as the antioxidant defense system, which keeps unruly free radicals in check. Our antioxidant defense system is brilliantly designed to gobble up free radical offenders and also to prevent their formation, but we need to remember that in order to operate in top form, the defense system is highly dependent upon dietary sources of antioxidants. Some major antioxidants are manufactured inside cells, but even here they require dietary nutrients to build them and make them effective.

For the most part, the antioxidant defense system helps things to run pretty smoothly. Problems arise, however, when the production of free radicals exceeds the capacity of the defense system, or when the defense system is running on low-quality dietary fuel. Significant quantities of dietary antioxidants are not found in fatty meat and simple carbohydrates like white flour; they are, however, found in large quantities in the very foods that are missing from the North American diet. Lack of dietary protection from fruits, vegetables, whole grains, fiber, and beneficial bacteria found in foods leads to cellular damage because the free radicals damage (oxidize) important components of our cells. Free radicals damage the fat and protein components of brain cells and, very importantly, they damage the genetic material, the DNA. In a vicious cycle, cellular damage actually leads to a greater generation of free radicals and therefore more cellular damage. While this is an inevitable part of aging and will happen to all of us eventually because the antioxidant defense system weakens with age, we don't have to sit idly by and watch it happen. Instead, we can take steps to minimize the genetic influences on aging and neurodegenerative conditions.

Dietary antioxidants can help put the brakes on the cellular damage and ensure optimal brain function not only in the distant future but also in the here and now. Oxidative stress and lack of dietary antioxidants is associated with decreased energy levels, and it also interferes with cognitive functioning. According to one of the largest reviews on the topic, published in the *Journal of Nutrition, Health and Aging* (2002), higher antioxidant status, reflected by blood levels of dietary antioxidants (e.g. vitamins C and E and beta-carotene), has been associated with enhanced memory function in older adults. Oxidative stress is now becoming recognized as a warning sign of later neurodegenerative diseases. In midlife, mild cognitive impairment is associated with higher levels of oxidative stress than in those with no measurable cognitive impairment.

There are a large number of brain-related conditions where oxidative stress is a common thread. As we will discuss, where there is oxidative stress there is usually also low-level chronic inflammation.

At present, scientists are unsure to what degree oxidative stress is a causative factor, or if it is really more of a consequence of brain-related conditions—perhaps it is both. Either way, the evidence connecting these brain conditions with increased generation of free radicals and diminished

**Neurological and Psychiatric Conditions
with Signs of Oxidative Stress**

Alzheimer's Disease	Chronic Fatigue Syndrome
Amyotrophic Lateral Sclerosis	Dementia
	Depression
Anxiety Disorders	Fibromyalgia
Attention Deficit Hyperactivity Disorder	Huntington's Disease
	Multiple Sclerosis
Autism	Schizophrenia

antioxidant protection is certainly not a good thing. Given that oxidative stress can damage cells, the generation of excess free radicals can have a detrimental effect on behavior and cognition by way of altered neuronal (brain cell) functioning. There are recent hints that oxidative stress may play a direct role in some mental conditions. Researchers writing in the prestigious journal *Nature* (2005) showed that over-expression of genes that turn on the antioxidant defense system in the brains of animals causes anxiety-related behaviors. In contrast, blocking the over-expression of these genes can decrease anxious behavior. This exciting new line of research provides a reason why there are signs of increased oxidative stress in anxiety disorders and other brain-related conditions.

It is entirely possible that the brain responds to the oxidative stress burden in our modern world by turning on the genes responsible for the production of the enzymes that ordinarily deal with oxidative stress—the problem being that these same genes when over-expressed (turned on too much) may be *negatively* influencing behavior in certain individuals. While drug companies spend millions, even billions, on drugs to influence genetics, a good starting point might be to turn up the antioxidant defense system by providing greater dietary antioxidant support—this will serve to combat the free radicals and may turn down the genetic over-expression. It is theoretical for now, but such influences of diet on genetic expression have been observed in other illnesses, most notably type II diabetes.

Research supports the notion that dietary antioxidants can influence brain cells and ultimately behavior in a positive way. As highlighted in a recent article in the *American Journal of Clinical Nutrition* (2005), researchers showed that antioxidants can not only prevent cognitive decline and neuronal dysfunction—blueberry in particular can reverse cognitive and behavioral deficits in experimental conditions; in addition to the antioxidant effects, the range of naturally occurring phytochemicals (including polyphenols) in blueberry might prevent and reverse cognitive and behavioral deficits by enhancing signaling between nerve cells. It appears that blueberry can make the nerve cell receptors friendlier toward binding with the brain's chemical messengers (neurotransmitters).

It's as if blueberry is the WD40® of the nerve cells. In one intriguing study, blueberry supplementation did not prevent the buildup of the characteristic beta-amyloid plaque in the animal model of Alzheimer's disease, but it did prevent the associated memory-related problems. Animals maintained on a blueberry-supplemented diet had higher levels of brain chemicals related to memory, even in the face of amyloid plaque buildup. These pigmented chemicals within blueberry and other dark berries appear to defy genetics.

There are additional benefits to blueberries, or at least the European variety called bilberry, in that they protect the tightly secured perimeter fence of the brain known as the blood-brain barrier. This is a specialized set of blood vessels that surround the brain; they are structurally different from other blood vessels because the brain cells are so incredibly delicate and require advanced protection from toxins. Phytochemicals from bilberry and grape seeds have been shown in research to prevent destruction of the blood-brain barrier by known toxins. This is of clinical relevance because conditions such as multiple sclerosis and chronic fatigue syndrome may be associated with an increased (and inappropriate) permeability of the barrier. A more porous blood-brain barrier may also be involved in the increased sensitivity to chemicals such as aspartame and monosodium glutamate as has been documented in fibromyalgia.

It is likely that many dietary antioxidants in addition to bilberry and grape seed work to keep the barrier working properly. Given the enormous amount and variety of manmade chemicals introduced into our environments and our diets, the maintenance of an intact blood-brain barrier becomes even more important. Keep in mind that stress, inflammation, infections, and cellular phone use may all cause a more porous blood-brain barrier. Dietary support of the blood-brain barrier is critically important in protecting the brain against environmental insults.

As exciting as the blueberry studies are (imagine such a delicious treat being so very beneficial!), they are absolutely not the whole story. They are only one instrument in the midst of a most amazing symphony orchestra of dietary antioxidants. We need not just blueberries but a host of different-colored fruits, vegetables, and culinary herbs. Within these plants are the phytochemicals that protect the brain. Searching for singular isolated nutrients that can prevent brain disorders has been a very disappointing hunting experience for neuroscientists. Studies with individual antioxidant supplements such as vitamin C and vitamin E have not been encouraging in neurological disorders, while studies using both together have yielded better results. The most solid research is in the area of dietary intake of foods containing vitamins C and E.

New research indicating that the sum of two antioxidants combined can be greater than that of the two parts added individually lends support to the idea that it is the synergy of the nutrients in whole foods that make them brain protective. This is also why I am not a fan of high levels, or so-called "megadoses," of individual antioxidant supplements. When you take very high doses of vitamin C or E alone, you are messing around with the sounds of the orchestra. Some antioxidants, like vitamin C, have a "bad boy" side and are actually capable of acting as a pro-oxidant and causing damage. Beta-carotene may have that Dr. Jekyll and Mr. Hyde effect also. A few studies have indicated that beta-carotene may act as a pro-oxidant in a way that actually promotes cancer in smokers when taken alone as a supplement. The good news is that taking antioxidants together can negate the potential pro-oxidant effects of individual antioxidants. In this case, the full orchestra covers up for the small mistake of one member—it goes unnoticed and the audience (your neurons) is thrilled with the results.

The Adequate Antioxidant Diet

The adequate antioxidant diet for brain health is pretty straightforward: simply meet the well-publicized and well-documented recommendations to eat five to ten servings of fruits and vegetables per day and you will be in excellent shape. Think variety and think deep colors. Five servings of iceberg lettuce and watermelon affords little protection for your brain cells, and fried potatoes, considered a vegetable serving, may actually do harm over time.

In order to take full advantage of the full benefits of the phytochemicals within plants, it is helpful to recognize some of the antioxidant super-stars. Nutrition scientists at the U.S. Department of Agriculture have identified the antioxidant values of more than 150 fruits, vegetables, berries, teas, nuts, spices, and prepared foods. Nutritional scientists rate antioxidant foods by the ORAC, or oxygen radical absorbance capacity, score. In essence, they look at the effectiveness of a food or nutrient in terms of its ability to handle and dispose of free radicals. A large portion of the Department of Agriculture's ongoing investigation into antioxi-dant foods was published in the *Journal of Agricultural and Food Chemistry* (2004). Some interesting findings emerged, including the observation that ORAC scores for apples are significantly higher with the peel on, that ORAC scores for some fruits are much higher in fresh and frozen forms than when canned in heavy syrup. A surprise to many was that nuts have very high ORAC scores and also of note is that a little spice goes a long way—cinnamon, cloves, mustard, and chili have tremendous antioxidant activity. Culinary herbs are also great: basil, oregano, and parsley, it turns out, are potent antioxidants.

If you have a passion for chocolate, you may be pleased to know that the dark variety, rich in cocoa, is a potent antioxidant food. Flavonoid-dense dark chocolate has been shown to have a beneficial effect on the cardiovascular system, lowering blood pressure, inhibiting the platelet activity that causes clots, and directly protecting blood vessels. Moder-ation is important with dark chocolate because it is also rich in calorie content. Interestingly, a study in the journal *Nutrition* (2005) showed that just the cocoa (without the added saturated fat) can actually lower body weight, fat cell (adipose tissue) weight, and triglycerides when incorpo-rated into an animal diet.

Sesame seeds are a wonderful antioxidant food that can specifically help to protect the fats that make up the walls of our cells. Sesame seeds contain a fibrous component called sesame lignans that can lower bad (LDL) cholesterol, help to enhance the antioxidant activity of vitamin E, and preserve the important omega-3 fatty acid levels. Dietary lignans have been linked to the preservation of cognitive functioning as we age.

Seaweeds are another highly nutritious food and a great source of antioxidants. New experimental research shows that seaweeds are actually protective of nerve cells. Sesame and seaweeds, scarcely consumed by North Americans at all, are widely consumed by the longest living peoples in the world, the Japanese. At least three studies have shown that black sesame seeds, popular in Japan, are even more effective than white sesame at protecting cells against free radical damage. Black sesame seeds and ground black sesame paste for entrées, baked goods, and smoothies are available at Asian grocery stores and at www.kenkonutrition.com.

Consider also that when researchers from Spain were examining the role of various foods in either enhancing or protecting us from damage to the fatty components of our cells, they were shocked to find that white potatoes were associated with increased oxidative stress. Writing in the *Journal of the American Dietetic Association* (2003), Cristina Lasheras reported that other forms of starches, such as rice and pasta, were not associated with such increases in oxidative damage to cells. Americans overconsume the white potato, a vegetable that offers only marginal levels of vitamins and minerals and clearly lacks the colorful phytochemicals found in orange sweet potatoes and Japanese purple sweet potatoes. An oven-roasted sweet potato complete with skin, known as *satsumaimo*, is a traditional snack for Japanese children, and certainly a healthy alternative to cake and candy. We all know how white potatoes are often served up to North Americans—fried without skins.

A glass or two of red wine appears to be brain protective and an excellent source of antioxidants. The concern, though, is with all the talk

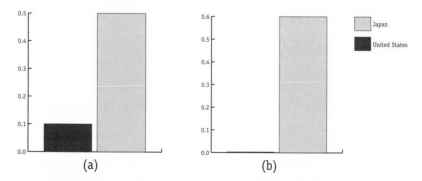

(a) Sesame seed consumption in kilograms per person, 2002; (b) Seaweed consumption in kilograms per person, 2002.

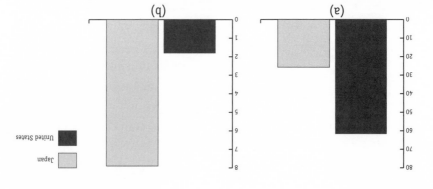

(a) White potato consumption in kilograms per person, 2002; (b) Sweet potato consumption in kilograms per person, 2002.

of how good some wines and other forms of alcohol are for health, it can be interpreted to mean that a little more might be even better. I need to point out that when larger quantities of alcohol are consumed over long periods of time, there are significant consequences to the brain. The effects include damage to the emotional center of the brain, the limbic system, and also to the memory center, the hippocampus. Even short-term binge drinking has been associated with damage to nerve cells and inhibition of the normal nerve cell development and growth that occurs in adulthood. Researchers from Germany found that red grape juice antioxidants were better absorbed than red wine, and in a 2005 study from Brazil, researchers concluded that purple grape juice may protect against coronary artery disease without the additional negative effects of alcohol.

Inflammation

Only a decade ago inflammation was synonymous only with arthritis or other conditions that ended in "-itis." That has certainly changed; in today's scientific world, inflammation has been associated with a host of human conditions, including heart disease, diabetes, obesity, and, yes, even neuropsychiatric conditions. On the cover of a recent *Time* magazine (February 23, 2004), inflammation earned its place in history as it was referred to as "The Secret Killer." Indeed, chronic inflammation wreaks havoc throughout the body and particularly in the brain. Why is inflammation the plague of the twenty-first century? As you

The HIGH ORAC Superstars—Major Dietary Brain-Friendly Antioxidants

Acai	Broccoli	High-quality olive	Prunes
Alfalfa	Brussels sprouts	oil	Purple cauliflower
Apple vinegar	Cherries	Kale	Purple sweet
Applesauce	Chili powder	Nuts (esp. walnuts,	potato
Artichoke	Cilantro	pecans, and	Raisins
Asparagus	Cinnamon	hazelnuts)	Raspberry
Avocado	Cloves	Oatmeal and *whole*	Red cabbage
Basil	Cocoa	*grain* breakfast	Red grapes
Beans (red, pinto,	Cranberry	cereals	Red leaf lettuce
black, navy)	Dates	Oranges	Red potatoes
Beets	Eggplant	Oregano	Spinach
Bell peppers	Elderberry	Parsley	Strawberry
Black-eyed peas	Figs	Peaches	Tangerines
Black pepper	Fuji apples	Pears	Turmeric
Blackberry	Ginger	Plums	
Blueberry	Green tea	Pomegranate	

may have guessed, the Western diet, with its trans and saturated fats and its sedentary context, is the biggest contributor to the inflammation plague. Lack of dietary antioxidants has also been shown to promote inflammation, and in turn, a state of chronic inflammation uses up precious antioxidants.

Chronic inflammation is provoked by excess intake of saturated fats and by excess dietary sugars. In addition, our overconsumption of omega-6 fatty acids (e.g. corn, safflower, soybean, and sunflower oils) has been shown in many studies to promote inflammation. Together, saturated fats, trans fats, and excess omega-6 fatty acids encourage the production of inflammatory chemicals called prostaglandins, particularly the series-2 type called PGE2. These fats also direct the production of immune chemicals called cytokines, which can really do a number on mood, cognition, and long-term brain health.

What is so important about these cytokines? Consider a study in the *Archives of General Psychiatry* (2001) where healthy adults were administered a small amount of a toxin that promotes the production of inflammatory cytokines; researchers discovered that these healthy adults had three major complaints as a result of cytokine elevations . . . depression, anxiety, and cognitive complaints! A host of animal studies have shown a similar effect of cytokine elevations on behavior and cognition in various laboratory settings. The bottom line is that these chemicals can have acute effects on how we feel and how sharply we think.

Over the long haul, chronic inflammation begins to wear down delicate brain cells, and it is responsible for actual structural damage to the nerve cells. Chronic inflammation provokes the manufacture of the senile plaques and neuro-fibrillary tangles observed in Alzheimer's disease. At least twenty published studies have shown a protective effect of anti-inflammatory agents against the development of Alzheimer's disease. Long term use of anti-inflammatories has been shown to reduce the risk of Alzheimer's disease by 60 to 80 percent and Parkinson's disease by as much as 45 percent. Dietary influences on the development and progression of neurological and psychiatric conditions has, until very recently, been underappreciated.

The Anti-Inflammatory Diet

Many fruits, vegetables, and culinary herbs have tremendous anti-inflammatory properties; ultimately, the anti-inflammatory diet is a diet high in antioxidants as well because the two go hand in hand. Antioxidants have been shown to lower inflammatory markers in humans. We will take a closer look at the effects of fish and omega-3 fatty acid supplements in the next chapter. Just remember that fish, particularly oily ocean fish (salmon, sardines, mackerel, anchovy), is the most potent anti-inflammatory food you can put into your body. Canola oil, walnuts, and ground flaxseeds are also important sources of the anti-inflammatory omega-3 fatty acid. More on this in the next chapter. Now let's have a look at some anti-inflammatory brain-protective superstars.

TURMERIC

Otherwise known as *Curcuma longa*, this is the yellow powder found in curry, and in a number of experimental studies it has been shown to have significant neuroprotective and mood-enhancing properties. Among the active chemicals in this root is a chemical called curcumin. This is an absolutely brilliant plant antioxidant and has significant anti-inflammatory properties. At least four human studies have shown that curcumin can decrease inflammation, and a host of studies show that it can specifically inhibit the mood- and cognition-disrupting cytokines.

Where curcumin really exerts its authority is protecting the mito-chondria in the nerve cells. The mitochondria are the energy packets of the cell, and you can imagine them as little AA batteries. When these lit-tle houses of energy, the mitochondria, are functioning in subpar fashion, so too will the entire nervous system. To make matters worse, when the mitochondria are damaged, there is increased generation of those free radical "thugs." They, in turn, beat up on an already weak and shaky mitochondria. Turmeric comes to the rescue and has been shown to cut off this cycle. It is interesting to note that the daily average intake of cur-cumin is negligible in North America, while in India, where rates of Alzheimer's disease are much lower, it is between 60 and 100 mg per day.

Incredible new experimental research published in the *Journal of Biological Chemistry* (2005) shows that not only does turmeric prevent the buildup of the amyloid plaque characteristic of Alzheimer's, in aged ani-mals turmeric actually breaks up the plaque. While curcumin makes up only 4 percent of the total chemical composition of turmeric, it packs a powerful punch. In animal experiments published in the *European Journal of Pharmacology* (2005) and the *Journal of Ethnopharmacology* (2002), turmeric has been shown to exert an antidepressant effect under stressful conditions. In these experimental studies, the behavioral effects of turmeric were comparable to the antidepressant drug fluoxetine (Prozac). Turmeric can help prevent the breakdown of important neurotransmit-ters, particularly mood-regulating serotonin and dopamine. It is antici-pated that researchers will begin to specifically examine curcumin for an antidepressant effect in humans. The research on turmeric and curcumin indicates that it is one of those minor dietary elements that can influence genetic expression, which, as stated already, means that it can ultimately influence the onset and/or progression of disease. Exciting new research in the *Journal of Neuroinflammation* (2005) shows that curcumin can specifically inhibit the production of inflammatory brain chemicals at the genetic level. Combine that with the other animal studies showing that curcumin decreases oxidative damage and reverses plaque-related cogni-tive deficits, and turmeric emerges as a star. If that is not enough for you, then consider this eye-opening study published in the *Annals of the New York Academy of Sciences* (2004) where mice fed tetrahydrocurcumin had an increased life expectancy of 125.9 percent over animals fed standard laboratory chow. Tetrahydrocurcumin is a metabolite, or breakdown product, of curcumin, and it has a more significant antioxidant activity than curcumin alone. Of course this doesn't mean that tetrahydrocurcumin is the fountain of youth, but it should encourage you to spice up your plate a little!

GINGER

It is not entirely surprising that ginger would also have significant anti-inflammatory and neuroprotective properties, given that turmeric and ginger are in the same plant family. Ginger has a 2,500-year history of traditional use in India and China as a medicinal agent, particularly for headaches and gastrointestinal complaints. Much like turmeric, ginger has many active chemicals, and researchers have focused in on gingerol for its medicinal properties. There is no question that ginger is an anti-inflammatory agent; this idea is supported not only by animal studies, but also in at least four human studies as well. The gingerols have been shown to specifically inhibit inflammatory chemicals of neuropsychiatric significance.

Ginger is also one of those minor nutritional players that can pack a major genetic punch. Researchers from RMG Biosciences in Baltimore, Maryland, showed for the first time in late 2004 that ginger can influence the manufacture of inflammatory brain chemicals at the genetic level. Ginger therefore has the potential to delay the onset of and slow down the progression of brain conditions associated with inflammation. Previous research has shown that ginger also has anti-anxiety properties in animals and reduces oxidative stress in the brain of laboratory animals. Ginger specifically protects the fat components of the nerve walls against free radical attack. According to research published in *Neurobiology of Aging* (2002), when combined with ginkgo biloba, ginger can prevent the expected age-related declines in mental performance. Liberal use of ginger and turmeric is encouraged, as both should be considered bodyguards for nerve cells and both can put out the flames of inflammation.

GREEN TEA

Research shows that regular consumption of green tea has multiple health benefits. Green tea contains a blend of phytochemicals called catechins, which are potent antioxidants with significant anti-inflammatory properties. In particular, epigallocatechin-3-gallate (EGCG) is a key player among the catechins, and it is known to dampen down those inflammatory chemicals called cytokines and prostaglandins.

Green tea consumption has been shown to lower cholesterol and blood pressure and decrease the risk of stroke. A recent Japanese study in *Circulation Journal* (2004) showed that green tea consumption is directly related to a lowered risk of coronary artery disease. Green tea inhibits the growth of potentially harmful bacteria, yet incredibly, it promotes the growth of beneficial intestinal bacteria—*Lactobacillus* and *Bifidobacteria*. As we will discuss in chapter 6, this attribute of green tea is a very, very good thing.

A growing body of research shows that green tea has properties that make it a strong candidate in the prevention of damage to nerve cells characteristic of such conditions as Alzheimer's and Parkinson's diseases. A recent experimental study in the *Journal of Immunology* (2004) indicates that the combined anti-inflammatory and brain-cell protecting properties of green tea shows promise for the prevention and treatment of multiple sclerosis. The synergistic actions of the catechins exert powerful antioxidant activity and protect the brain cells against the effects of aging. Recent human studies also show that green tea, and EGCG in particular, can assist in the reduction of abdominal fat.

In addition to the long-term benefits, sipping some green tea can provide an immediate lift in mood and mental focus due to the low levels of caffeine and an amino acid called L-theanine, which has relaxing effects. The Japanese have been enjoying green tea as part of their traditional diet for years. The highest grade of green tea is Japanese *matcha*—a fine powder of the finest green tea leaves. In 2003, researchers from the University of Colorado found that the concentration of EGCG available from drinking matcha is up to 137 times greater than the amount of EGCG available from other commercially available green teas. (See www.kenkonutrition.com for premium matcha powder from Japan.) This matcha can not only be used to make the traditional hot beverage, small amounts can also be incorporated into baked goods and smoothies.

There is some concern from experimental studies that green tea may induce a deficiency of the B vitamin folic acid by its inhibition of an enzyme involved in folate metabolism. Therefore, if you are drinking more than a couple of cups of green tea a day or taking green tea supplements, then taking a folic acid supplement may be advisable.

NUTS

Until recently, nuts were unfairly dismissed as a fat-laden dietary item that should be avoided. After some solid scientific research, nuts have emerged as nutritional superstars. They provide us with the good mono- and polyunsaturated fats, vitamin E, heart-healthy compounds called sterols, and anti-inflammatory components, and they also pack a potent antioxidant punch. Consuming nuts at least twice a week has been associated with significant reductions in the risk of dying from coronary heart disease. The decreased risk is not small; the numbers are dramatic and run from 35 to 50 percent, depending on the study population. In intervention studies where individuals are given nuts to eat over time, researchers consistently see a lowering of the bad (LDL) cholesterol.

In addition to heart health, new research by neuroscientists from the University of Illinois–Chicago showed that nuts, and almonds in particular, prevent age-induced mental decline. Specifically, in addition to normal chow, almonds were added to one group of mice with the early stages of Alzheimer's disease. The mice taking almonds for four months performed much better on memory tests than the animals in the standard chow group. The animals consuming the human equivalent of about a handful of almonds per day also had a reduction in the abnormal plaque deposits associated with Alzheimer's disease.

Despite the fear that nuts are calorie-dense and consumption will cause weight gain, research has actually shown that those who moderately consume nuts on a regular basis weigh less than those who do not. Intervention studies also indicate that participants consuming nuts do not gain the expected weight due to increased nut intake, and although much more research is needed, it appears that nuts are more satiating and may increase the use of fat as an energy source. The key is moderation: a palm sized, or 1-ounce, serving as a snack that would otherwise be a donut, margarine-based muffin, or Danish is the way to go. Walnuts are a significant source of anti-inflammatory omega-3 fatty acids and they also contain the sleep-regulating and potent antioxidant chemical called melatonin. Almonds, pecans, pistachios, and peanuts all have scientific research to support consumption as a heart-healthy dietary choice. When it comes to the health of the brain, any item that can keep blood flowing to the brain while delivering important antioxidants and healthy fats is a good choice.

PURPLE/DEEP RED FOODS

Foods that contain purple-colored pigments called anthocyanins are now being recognized as extra special when it comes to protecting our blood vessels and our nerve cells. Examples of such foods include blueberries, bilberries (European blueberry), dark cherries, purple carrots (yes, they come in purple too!), pomegranate, acai, purple sweet potatoes, purple cauliflower, black grapes, and beets. The purple pigments offer significant antioxidant protection, enhance signaling between nerve cells, protect the blood-brain barrier, and strengthen the blood vessels that supply blood to the brain. If you need still more convincing, they have also been shown to exert a significant anti-inflammatory effect capable of reducing pain. The purple sweet potato is immensely popular as a health food in Japan, where it is one of the dietary contributors reported to assist in healthy longevity. The extract of this purple spud has found its way into health drinks in Japan and North America.

GREEN FOODS

A few years ago in Toronto I was shocked to see a nutritionally offensive billboard from a Canadian fast-food chain—it was a huge close up picture of a massive burger on a bun with the words "Greens are for golf." I beg to differ. Dark green vegetables of all sorts contain a precious mineral that can quench the flames of inflammation. That mineral, worth its weight in nutritional gold, is called magnesium. The green pigment of plants is called chlorophyll, and magnesium makes up an important part of this chemical found in nature's greens. Over half of the U.S. population does not meet even the minimum recommendations for daily intake of magnesium. The fact that we fall short on daily servings of fruits and vegetables probably has much to do with that reality. In a study published in the *Journal of the American College of Nutrition* (2005), researchers from the Medical University of South Carolina showed that in almost four thousand adults, those with low dietary magnesium intake (50 percent RDA) were about three times more likely (versus those meeting the RDA) to have levels of C-reactive protein that are in the danger zone. What is this C-reactive protein? It has long been recognized as a blood marker of

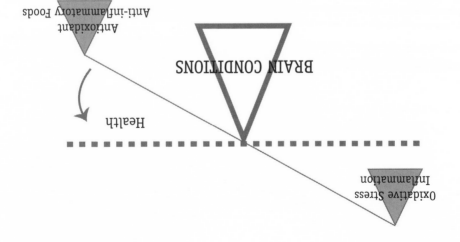

inflammation, but more recently doctors have been making some major connections between elevations in this inflammatory marker and the risk of dying from cardiovascular disease. In fact, a recent study showed C-reactive protein to be a better predictor of coronary heart disease than bad (LDL) cholesterol. This is important because more than 50 percent of those who die from coronary heart disease have normal cholesterol levels. It also turns out that C-reactive protein is elevated in cases of depression and panic disorder, and it is now linked to neurological conditions.

Incredibly, the low-carb nonsense that swept the United States in 2002 actually discouraged liberal consumption of magnesium containing vegetables because they are carbs! With that in mind, you may not be surprised to know that when researchers from Virginia Polytechnic Institute and State University put a group of adults on a low-carb diet similar to that of Atkins, the end result was elevated levels of C-reactive protein. Bottom line—eat your greens for your heart and your brain.

Sugar and Inflammation—The AGE Connection

There is no question that we consume way too much dietary sugar in North America. Excess sugar leads to blood sugar abnormalities and an increased risk of obesity, neurological conditions, and depression. Diabetes is becoming an established risk factor for Alzheimer's disease, and now neuropsychiatric connections are also being made with chronically elevated blood sugar. Consider the eye-opening research published in the journal *Depression and Anxiety* (2002), which showed a clear connection between higher rates of sugar consumption and higher rates of depression among nations. In Japan, where rates of depression are much lower than North America, the annual consumption of sugar and sweeteners is less than half that of the United States and Canada.

With excess sugar floating around, there is greater glycation, the fancy name for the attachment of sugars to proteins. Glycation, also called the

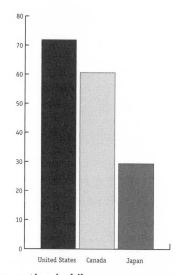

Sugar consumption in kilograms per person, 2002.

Maillard reaction, is initiated by the addition of sugar to proteins, and it ends up producing, after a series of reactions, advanced glycation end products (AGEs). Glycation wreaks havoc—it leads to the production of damaging free radicals and promotes inflammation. Aptly named AGEs alter the structure and physiological activities of proteins. Once this happens, there is interference with the lines of communication among nerve cells and disturbances inside those cellular energy factories called mitochondria. To make matters worse, oxidative stress promotes the formation of AGEs and so the cycle continues. Glycation and AGEs have been associated with various brain conditions, including Alzheimer's disease, Parkinson's disease, and amyotrophic lateral sclerosis (ALS). Given the connection with oxidative stress, it is realistic to assume that AGEs are associated with many neuropsychiatric conditions.

The world's leading authority on glycation and its long-term effects on the nervous system is Dr. Seiji Kikuchi of Hokkaido University in

Sapporo, Japan. His team has shown that the components of glycation are indeed present in the central nervous system of ALS patients. As he suggests in the journal *Brain Research Reviews* (2003), glycation will not lead to damage to neurons overnight; rather, it is a slow process that advances over time. However, it can and does catch up with us as we age, particularly in those with genetic susceptibilities.

So we now know that AGEs are toxic to nerve cells and we know that they promote inflammation and oxidative stress. We also know that overconsumption of dietary sugar plays a role. The question is, of course, how can we cut off this vicious cycle? Obviously, we need first and foremost to lower our intake of added sugar and sweeteners. Soft drinks, candies, cakes, ice cream, cookies, etc., will spike the blood sugar levels and promote AGE formation. It should also be noted that some foods are themselves a direct source of AGEs. A number of dietary items contain high levels of AGEs that form during cooking and processing. Specifically, oven- and deep-frying food is not a good idea if you want to keep your AGE intake to a minimum. Poaching, steaming, and boiling are much better options. The presence of moisture helps keep AGEs formed in cooking to a minimum. Dietary values of AGEs are expressed in kilounits (ku), and with that in mind consider that a 90 g serving of chicken breast provides 9000 ku when it is oven-fried. That number drops dramatically to 5,250 ku when the same serving is prepared using the broiler. A roast chicken is even better at 4300 ku and a boiled chicken (as found in a soup) only has 1000 ku of AGE. Butter has double the the AGE content of a comparable serving of olive oil.

Some processed food requires high and dry heat (over 230°C), which can help to explain why commercial snack foods, waffles, and cookies have extraordinary AGE values per serving. Consider that a 30 g serving of vanilla biscotti has a whopping 966 ku of AGE, more than double that of an oatmeal raisin cookie of similar weight. Also, I hate to break this to you, but if you want to maintain optimal brain functioning and cognition, you will have to avoid hot dogs. Next time you are out at the ballpark, stop and think about your brain cells before you and the kids consume an incredible 10,143 ku of AGE in just one 90 g serving of frankfurter! Research shows that dietary restriction of high-AGE foods and instructions on using boiling and stewing versus deep frying and high-dry heat leads to a dramatic reduction in AGEs circulating in the bloodstream. Perhaps most importantly, a low dietary AGE plan is associated with significant reductions in inflammatory chemicals at the genetic level. Incorporating a low-AGE diet by avoiding high-AGE foods and utilizing boiling, stewing, poaching, and steaming will go a long way toward preserving your brain cells and lowering oxidative stress and inflammation. Given that AGE promotes oxidative stress, a diet high in antioxidants can also help to cut off the cycle. As you know, the high-antioxidant diet is full of a variety of colorful fruits and vegetables, whole grains, and oils with minimal processing. In addition to this, there are some dietary supplements that show promise as AGE inhibitors. Turmeric, a brain-protecting, antioxidant amino acid, has been shown in a recent study to prevent excessive glycation and the accumulation of AGEs in animals fed a high-sugar diet.

Carnosine, a dipeptide formed naturally in human tissues, is maintained at high levels in long-lived cells such as those in the brain (neurons). The concentration of carnosine in tissue correlates with maximum life span, which suggests it is a potential biomarker of longevity. Carnosine is now available as a dietary supplement and may help put a significant dent in glycation, particularly when combined with taurine and/or alpha-lipoic acid (ALA). New research suggests that ALA can inhibit the action of AGEs. ALA is an antioxidant superstar because it works as both a water-soluble and water-insoluble scavenger of free radicals. Last, but certainly not least, a recent review in the journal *Biogerontology* (2004) by glycation experts from the University of Mumbai, India, has highlighted the potential benefits of B vitamins (thiamine and B6), vitamins C and E, and green tea as AGE inhibitors.

It is important to note that a supplement containing 50 to 100 mg of carnosine is not going to have much of an effect on human AGE at all because ingested carnosine is acted upon by enzymes and is degraded rapidly. Based on published studies, the scientists at the Life Extension Foundation have recommended 1000 mg of carnosine in order to maintain relevant blood levels. The Life Extension Foundation is an organization dedicated to investigating every method of extending the healthy human life span; they have clearly been ahead of the curve when it comes to nutritional influences on aging brains. The medical and scientific advisory board of the Life Extension Foundation consists of a dream team of fifty leading experts in anti-aging medicine. See the Appendix for more

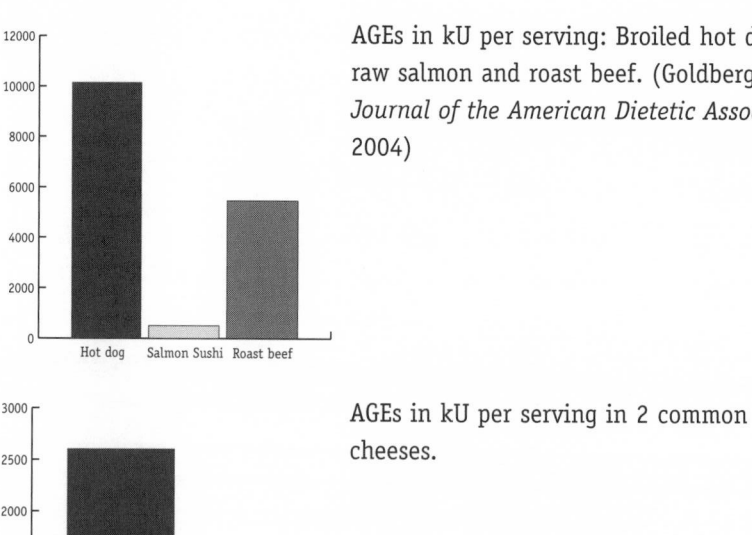

AGEs in kU per serving: Broiled hot dog, raw salmon and roast beef. (Goldberg et al. *Journal of the American Dietetic Association,* 2004)

AGEs in kU per serving in 2 common cheeses.

What's for breakfast? AGEs in kU per serving in 3 common breakfast options.

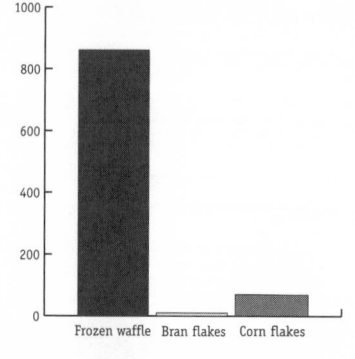

Snack, anyone? AGEs in kU per serving of some snack options.

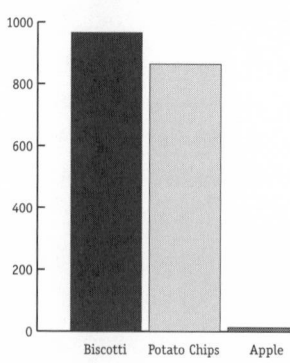

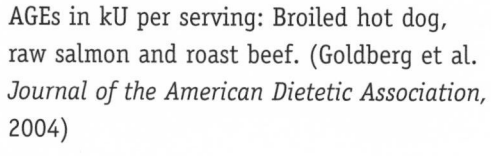

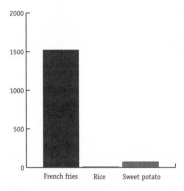

Side dish, anyone? AGEs in kU per serving of some side dishes: French fries, boiled rice, or an oven roasted sweet potato.

details on Life Extension's carnosine formulations.

Lots to Love about Starbucks

When it comes to human health, there are lots of reasons to love a good cup of coffee. Worldwide coffeehouses are filled every day with people from all walks of life, many of whom converge on these modern social centers for more than just a great cup of java. If you ever sit and just look around a Starbucks you will see future scientists studying hard, business executives closing deals, teenagers talking about the future, artists and performers discussing a show, and the elderly smiling about their new plans. Some sit alone, simply to get away from life for a little while. There is an abundance of research on the benefits of social support and enjoyable human interactions on health . . . but there is also an important benefit of coffeehouses within the context of the Brain Diet . . . the direct health *benefits* of coffee and low to moderate caffeine intake on the human brain.

For years coffee and caffeine have had an undeserved bad reputation. In fact, the myth that moderate coffee consumption is bad for you is just

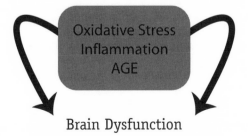

Cycle of Destruction: Oxidative stress, inflammation and accelerated AGE formation are central to most brain-related conditions. The Brain Diet plan can help to cut off this cycle.

that—a myth. Coffee contains a host of naturally occurring chemicals, including potent antioxidants. Coffee is so rich in beneficial phytochem-icals that it was stated in a recent study in the *Journal of Agricultural and Food Chemistry* (2004) that "coffee contains many antioxidants and con-sumption of antioxidant-rich coffee may inhibit diseases caused by oxida-tive damage." The study, a joint effort by Dr. Kenichi Yanagimoto of the University of California at Davis and colleagues from the Japan Institute for the Control of Aging, showed that coffee is particularly effective at protecting the fat component of cells against oxidative stress. Given that the brain is 60 percent fat, you may not be surprised to learn that coffee consumption has been associated with a lower risk of neurodegenerative diseases, including Alzheimer's and Parkinson's diseases. These findings in human epidemiological studies are supported by animal studies where coffee and low to moderate caffeine use reduce neurotoxicity. A cup or two of coffee is a pretty neat way to get in a daily fix of antioxidants, espe-cially when you consider that moderate doses of caffeine, 100–200 mg daily, are associated with increased energy, well-being, self-confidence, social disposition, motivation for work, and endurance. So unlike some other antioxidants, where you may not feel the immediate effects, coffee provides a little mood boost.

Consider that when 130,000 persons were followed over eight years, those who consumed more coffee were less likely to die by suicide. A sep-arate study found that in female Japanese medical students, coffee con-sumption was associated with fewer depressive symptoms. If you still want more, consider that coffee has been associated with a 30 percent decrease in the risk of diabetes, and lifetime consumption is associated with the maintenance of cognitive function later in life and a decreased risk of liver disease, colon cancer, and gallstones. A number of anti-caffeine and anti-coffee Web sites report that caffeine causes osteoporosis because it increases calcium elimination from the body and prevents its absorption. Most population studies have found no relationship between coffee or tea and osteoporosis, and a leading authority on bone health, Dr. Robert Heaney of Creighton University, reported in the journal *Food and Chemical Toxicology* (2002) that there is no evidence of a detrimental effect as long as an individual meets daily calcium requirements.

Now that scientists have uncovered some of the beneficial antioxi-dant chemicals within coffee, its contribution to overall dietary antioxi-

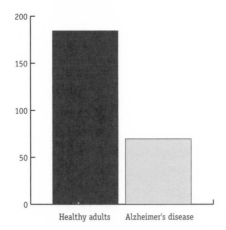

Average caffeine in mg consumed by twenty-five- to fifty-year-olds in the time span covering twenty to fifty years before diagnosis of Alzheimer's disease. (Maia, et al. *European Journal of Neurology*, 2002)

dant intake has become better appreciated. This was highlighted recently in a Norwegian study in the *Journal of Nutrition* (2004), where to the surprise of the investigators, the single greatest contributor to the total dietary antioxidant intake was indeed coffee, and the same number one slot for coffee was recently reported for the United States. Additional research in the *European Journal of Clinical Nutrition* (2003) shows that in Spain, coffee is the number one beverage contributing to total antioxidants in the diet, about three times higher than that of red wine.

The saying "everything in moderation" is of course also true of coffee and overall caffeine intake. Typically, just a cup or two of coffee confers benefits, but there are some individuals on this planet who were just not meant to drink coffee. A small minority of healthy adults are particularly sensitive to caffeine. Individuals with anxiety disorders including panic and social phobia, those with insomnia, and in general people with mental disorders should take great care in evaluating whether or not low to moderate caffeine intake might exacerbate symptoms. This note should be taken seriously, as research shows that the negative influence of caffeine on the course of various mental disorders is often overlooked by both patients and providers. Thankfully, decaffeinated coffees and teas are available, beverages that still provide significant antioxidant support.

For those who don't care for the taste of coffee, then tea, and green tea in particular, can also provide neuroprotective plant chemicals . . .

and while they don't have pure Japanese matcha (yet), you can get a great cup of green tea at Starbucks! Stick with low fat when it comes to adding milk to coffee or when asking for latte, and keep your green tea plain without sugar. It goes without saying that green tea or coffee-based drinks that are simply high-fat milkshakes are not brain friendly—they are for occasional use only. Also, these so-called energy drinks that have taken North America by storm are very high in sugar, almost 30 grams in a small 250 ml can. Researchers have recently suggested that these drinks may contribute to tooth decay and obesity.

The Brain Diet and Cell Phones

I'm often asked about the safety of cellular phones. It is clear that cellular phones, in just a few short years of existence, have changed the way we live. They are part of our culture, and there is no question that they can be the most convenient little device ever made, not to mention being a life-saver in emergency situations. Many people have a love-hate relationship with cell phones—they love their own and hate when other people use them. The number of U.S. cell phone subscribers is inching close to 200 million, and there are more than 175,000 cell phone towers dotted over the American landscape. The explosion in cell phone use occurred in the late 1990s. As prices have dropped, the number of minutes used by Americans has skyrocketed—collectively, we now spend more than four trillion minutes per year talking on cell phones.

As intrusive and annoying cell phone conversations and ring tones in public places may be, it is the disturbing research on the effects of microwave radiation that is relevant to brain health. In various parts of the world, a handful of scientists have been raising red flags concerning cellular phones over the past few years. As Dr. Leif Salford of the University of Lund, Sweden, stated in a recent issue of *Environmental Health Perspectives* (2003), cell phones have become the largest biologic experiment ever to be conducted in the history of humanity. He and his colleagues found that cell phone–type exposure is capable of causing nerve cell damage in the brains of mammals. His group has shown that electromagnetic fields similar to those of current cell phones can significantly open up the perimeter fence around the brain called the blood-brain barrier. This could be a real problem for those concerned about

• • • CASE REPORT • • •

Dan is a thirty-nine-year-old investment banker. He reported significant stress at home and in the workplace. Like many North Americans, he felt that the stress of the daily grind interfered with his quality of life. His chief complaint was insomnia, and he sought a natural approach to improve his sleep.

Dan's diet was actually quite good—well-balanced and inclusive of a variety of fruits and vegetables. He was appreciative of his wife, who made every effort to ensure the family was eating well. The problem captured on a diet diary was excessive caffeine intake, equal to six cups of coffee per day. In addition, Dan relied upon additional caffeine in the form of commercial energy drinks and cola.

The primary objective was to lower the perception of stress and strengthen Dan's coping abilities. Dan began using the relaxation response developed by Dr. Herbert Benson of Harvard Medical School. Every morning and night, Dan set aside just ten minutes to concentrate on his chosen word or phrase while in a relaxed state. Within a few weeks, Dan was able to use the relaxation response in times of stress, cutting off the cycle of stress hormones. He also became more mindful, reserved judgments, and made every effort to stay in the present. Dan became less "reactive" to stress, and this enhanced his perception of his own ability to cope. Using the mind-body approaches made him more resilient to stress.

Dan cut back on caffeine as well—within a few weeks he had it down to two cups of coffee and two cups of green tea per day, spaced out nicely and with 4:00 p.m. the "last call" for caffeine. Like many adults with insomnia, he had overlooked his evening coffee as a factor in sleep quality. Dan began to take a nightcap of a powdered milk protein containing high levels of alpha-lactalbumin (ALA). ALA is the component of milk known to boost serotonin levels; new research shows that ALA has a stress-buffering effect and helps to enhance sleep. Inadequate dietary magnesium may also be part of poor sleep, so 300 mg of magnesium citrate was taken along with a multivitamin at the evening meal. Dan was delighted with his improved sleep, mental focus at work, and overall quality of life.

keeping toxins out of the vicinity of brain tissue. The function of a tight blood-brain barrier is to exclude toxins. The opening of the barrier and type of nerve cell damage observed by Dr. Salford and his colleagues may not have clinical consequences for years. In effect, we may be setting the stage for a generation of cell phone users who may experience early onset of neurodegenerative diseases such as Alzheimer's.

In 2004, Turkish researchers showed that exposure to the equivalent of about one hour of mobile phone use could increase oxidative stress within the mammalian brain. Cell phones as a source of additional oxidative stress becomes a real concern in those with brain conditions, particularly with our lack of dietary antioxidant protection. In the United Kingdom, the National Radiological Protection Board (government advisory board) has urged parents to restrict the use of cellular phones in children.

Meanwhile, an article in the *San Francisco Chronicle* (February 27, 2005) reports that some teens carry two cell phones, one for local and one for long distance, and that cell phones are "more important than a nutritious meal"! This is double trouble—a young person exposed to a device that may increase oxidative stress in the brain combined with a lack of nutritional antioxidant protection. Clearly, this may set the stage for long-term problems.

According to the Spanish Neuro-Diagnostic Research Institute, it takes only two minutes on a cell phone to cause significant changes in brain activity, and an opening of the blood-brain barrier in children. The long-term effects of cellular phones on mood, learning, and attention have not been investigated. Based on the new Spanish research, which showed that microwaves from cell phones penetrate the brain more deeply than expected, altering natural electrical brain activity, it would not be a surprising if they altered cognition and behavior. The researchers are reported to have found that a two-minute cell phone call altered brain activity for up to an hour after the call ended. Cell phones may also influence sleep quality when left by the bedside.

Another huge question surrounding cell phones is the effect on so-called "innocents." Cell phones are now being compared to secondhand smoke in terms of exposure to nonusers. A non-cell phone user cannot control or avoid microwave radiation in certain public situations. World-renowned physicist Dr. Tsuyoshi Hondou of Tohoku University in Japan has recently debunked the notion that simply being away from a cell phone is protective. His formula, published in the *Journal of the Physical Society of Japan* (2002), demonstrates that in crowded places such as commuter trains, the effects of cell phones are additive and increase the potential risks of exposure.

Cell phones have been shown to negatively alter the short-term cognitive functions of adults, to increase oxidative stress in the brain, and to alter the levels of certain brain chemicals. In a nutshell, cell phones are a legitimate concern for medical scientists, but it is clear that this technology is not going anywhere. In a poll, 70 percent of teen users said they would not change the use of their phone even in the face of a government advisory. No one is going to turn off the big cell phone switch in the sky anytime soon—nor am I saying it should be turned off—even if there was one. For now, most international governments have accepted the short-term cell phone safety data and set exposure guidelines. However, no one can say at this point what, if any, long-term effects might start emerging from extended cell phone use. So, the real question for extensive users is, how can we protect our brains in a world where technology might be causing increased oxidative stress and an additional burden in a stressful world?

With that in mind, there is good news in that dietary antioxidants may prevent some of the potential negative consequences of cell phones, at least in animals. For instance, ginkgo biloba, a botanical medicine known for its role as a potent antioxidant and memory enhancer, has been shown to prevent oxidative damage induced by cellular phone exposure in animals. In addition, researchers from Turkey have consistently shown in a number of studies, the latest in *Archives of Medical Research* (2005) and *Molecular and Cellular Biochemistry* (2006), that the administration of melatonin and other antioxidants can prevent the oxidative stress induced by cell phones. Melatonin is a brain hormone (and dietary supplement) that is known to be a potent antioxidant.

While supplements, herbals, and other dietary items have not been investigated in terms of cell phone exposure in humans, the deeply colored pigments and phytochemicals from blueberries, bilberry, and grape seeds have been documented to protect against inappropriate opening of the blood-brain barrier and to prevent oxidative stress in living systems.

I'm not trying to be a scaremonger about this issue. There are lots of Internet sites set up simply to frighten the public into buying useless "protective" gizmos to attach to your phone. There are, however, legitimate concerns that need to be addressed. Given that cell phone–type exposure can increase oxidative stress within the brains of mammals, it means they have the potential to influence genetic expression and therefore may ultimately influence the onset and course of brain-related conditions. Remember, it's all about genetic susceptibility, and only time will uncover the consequences, if any, of our newfangled electromagnetic radiation exposure. The emerging research on cell phones should simply encourage you to maximize your intake of protective antioxidant nutrients. Protection comes not from the charlatans with pseudoscientific devices, crystals, and antenna gadgets purported to lower electromagnetic radiation—it comes from your diet rich in antioxidant foods.

Summary

When it comes to the long-term protection of your brain cells and the maintenance of optimal brain functioning, there are two common threads that must be cut off—oxidative stress and inflammation. The production and dietary ingestion of advanced glycation end products (AGEs) is another enemy within "the axis of neurotoxins." The excess production of free radicals and inflammatory chemicals can lead to acute alterations in mood and cognition; however, most often it goes undetected over years. The influence of inflammation and the generation of free radicals on neurological and psychiatric conditions is now the focus of international research. Whether cause or effect, or both, oxidative stress and inflammation can certainly contribute to the progression of brain-related conditions. The good news is that the human body can quench free radicals and hose down the fires of inflammation by dietary means.

Diets rich in colorful fruits and vegetables, whole grains, and oily fish can provide an abundance of antioxidants and healthy fats that can dampen inflammation. In addition, cooking methods that avoid deep frying and instead focus on steaming, poaching, boiling, and stewing can dramatically cut down the AGE chemicals that assault the brain cells. Avoidance of foods that are highly processed and full of added sweeteners will also help to lower the AGE burden. Include in your diet spices and herbs such as cinnamon, turmeric, and ginger, which can act as body guards for your nerve cells . . . and enjoy your cup of coffee or green tea, knowing that you are defending your brain.

3

Chewing the Right Fat

FOR YEARS, GOVERNMENT AND PROFESSIONAL dietetic organizations have made North Americans live in fear of fat. The fat phobia is reflected in the old Food Guide Pyramid, developed by the U.S. Department of Agriculture (USDA) and endorsed by the American Dietetic Association (ADA). When it comes to fats and oils, the ADA has for years been telling us to "enjoy just a bit from the tip"! The advice made absolutely no distinction between types of dietary fat, and until April 2005, when the new MyPyramid was unveiled, all fats were lumped together. The USDA's new MyPyramid does give advice on fat types; however, the fat contribution to the pyramid is barely noticeable. In fact, on the pyramid poster, fats and oils are not mentioned at the pyramid base as a main dietary category. Many consumers will continue to interpret this as meaning all fats are bad. The nutritional reality is that fats and oils are critically important in brain health—we just need to chew on the *right* fat.

Given that 60 percent of the human brain is made up of fat, and that different dietary fats can affect genetic expression within the brain in divergent ways, the influence of fats on brain performance and health cannot be overestimated. If you look at the Traditional Healthy Asian Diet Pyramid, you can see that it is *red* meat that we should enjoy "just a bit from the tip"! Fish and shellfish and vegetable oils are prioritized and

49

made distinct. In contrast, the U.S. pyramid shows meat as a general group in which fish falls. As we will discuss, fish and shellfish and certain dietary oils contain fats critical for human brain function. Consider that the longest living peoples on earth, the Japanese, take advantage of the good fats on the Traditional Healthy Asian Diet Pyramid; why shouldn't you?

The human genetic profile has remained constant over the past forty thousand years; however, the composition of our dietary fat intake has changed radically in just the last half-century. We have significantly increased our saturated and trans fat intake, while at the same time our consumption of omega-3 fatty acids has taken a serious plunge. The void of omega-3 is being filled by omega-6 rich corn, safflower, sunflower, and soybean oils. Omega-6 fats have found their way into our food supply at an excessive rate. Genetically we have been accustomed to an omega-6 to omega-3 ratio of close to 1:1, a far cry from the current ratio, which is at least 10 parts, and up to 20 parts, omega-6 for every omega-3. The

The traditional healthy Asian diet pyramid.

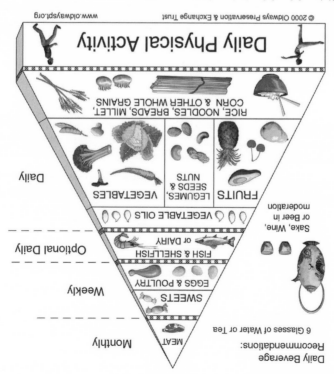

human brain, responsible for our civilization, art, music, science, architecture, and technology, has relied upon these important essential fatty acids, in proper balance, for at least the last forty millennia.

Remember that a diet top-heavy in omega-6 oils promotes inflammation and oxidative stress, both of which contribute to brain disorders. Excess saturated fats, and any amount of trans fat, can promote inflammation and alter the structure of the brain cells. Messing around with the evolution of dietary fat in a relatively short period of time is not without consequence. Brain structure and brain physiology can be dramatically altered, and cognition and behavioral disturbances are the end result. Depending on genetics, lifestyle, and experiences, a deficiency in omega-3 or an excess of other fats can lead to brain disorders.

Despite the omega-6 overload, some companies seem to ignore the research and actually incorporate omega-6-rich liquid sunflower oil and other cheap omega-6 oils into formulas. Knowing what we now know about the omega-6 saturation in the food supply, where is the scientific justification in supplementing North Americans with more of these oils? Worse still, sunflower and other omega-6-rich oils are mixed in with medium chain triglycerides (MCTs) in some commercial supplements. Incredible when you consider that MCTs, purported to increase energy, have been shown to raise cardiovascular risk in humans. The most recent study in the *American Journal of Clinical Nutrition* (2004) showed that MCT supplementation for twenty-one days led to significant increases in total cholesterol (11%), LDL cholesterol (12%), triglycerides (22%), and blood sugar (4%). Combining that with unnecessary omega-6 oils is clearly not a good thing, so be very, very cautious about so-called "best" commercial oil supplements, and be sure to check labels. I'll talk more about essential fatty acid supplements later.

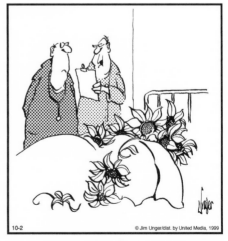

HERMAN®

10-2   © Jim Unger/dist. by United Media, 1999

"He'll be okay. He overdosed on sunflower seeds."

Conditions That Have Possible Connections to Low Omega-3 and/or Are Helped by Administration of Omega-3 Supplements

Alzheimer's disease/dementia	Borderline personality disorder	Huntington's disease
Social phobia	Childhood IQ/learning disorder	Migraine headaches
Attention deficit hyperactivity disorder (ADHD)	Chronic fatigue syndrome	Multiple sclerosis
Autism	Depression	Parkinson's disease
Bed-wetting (enuresis)	Dyslexia	Post-partum depression
Bipolar disorder	Dyspraxia	Schizophrenia
	Fibromyalgia	Seasonal affective disorder

To date, research has uncovered a significant connection between lower blood levels and lifetime intake of omega-3 fatty acids and both neurological and psychiatric conditions. In addition, the administration of omega-3 fatty acids has been found to be helpful in a number of conditions involving the brain.

Fats Influence Brain Genetics

We now know that the fats we eat are ultimately incorporated into the coating, or membrane, surrounding the nerve cell. The coating, scientifically known as the neuronal membrane, becomes hard and inflexible when there is excess saturated fat and not enough omega-3 in the wall (technically called the lipid bi-layer). Excess dietary cholesterol can also disturb the makeup of the lipid bi-layer in the neuronal membrane. This "hardening process" of the wall surrounding the nerve cell ultimately prevents proper signaling from nerve cell to nerve cell. The omega-3 fatty acids can not only displace cholesterol from the neuronal membrane and prevent its hardening, they are also responsible for signaling messengers that operate inside the nerve cells. Omega-3 fatty acids therefore are required for optimal signaling both between and within nerve cells.

A growing number of studies are demonstrating that omega-3 fatty acids can influence brain-related conditions at the genetic level. In rodent models of Alzheimer's and Huntington's disease, early and continuous treatment with omega-3 fatty acids protects against progression of the diseases, even in the presence of genetic susceptibilities. Omega-3 fatty acids can lower the oxidative stress and inflammation associated with neurological and psychiatric conditions, and very importantly, they can promote the genetic expression of a chemical known as brain derived neurotrophic factor (BDNF). This nerve growth factor plays a role in the growth, integrity, and survival of the developed, adult nervous system. Yes, believe it or not, brain development and nerve growth occurs even in adulthood.

BDNF is responsible for memory and cognition, and inhibition of BDNF neurogenesis (nerve growth) has been tied to many psychiatric and neurological conditions. Consider that low blood levels of BDNF are associated with more severe psychological depression. While you may think of nerve cell loss, damage, or shrinking mostly in neurological conditions, it is also evident in depression and other psychiatric conditions. BDNF is a potent neuroprotective agent, promoting the survival of nerve cells and optimal communication from cell to cell. It is no wonder that drug companies are spending millions to research medications that might influence or mimic BDNF. New research shows that expensive medications may not be necessary—BDNF can be influenced by lifestyle factors including exercise, avoiding saturated fats and too much sugar, and eating fish and/or taking inexpensive fish oil supplements.

I first suggested that omega-3 fatty acids can influence BDNF in the scientific literature in a well publicized article that appeared on *Medline* in November 2003. I suggested that omega-3 fatty acids could interfere with immune chemicals (cytokines) that prevent the manufacture of BDNF. I received scores of requests for my hypothesis from scientists located all over the globe. Researchers were as excited as I was—what if something as simple as fish fat could influence the levels of the billion-dollar chemical called BDNF? A year later, researchers from the UCLA confirmed that omega-3 fatty acids (a mixture of EPA and DHA) from fish oil can normalize BDNF levels in conditions of traumatic brain injury. Based on the mechanisms I outlined in 2003, EPA is likely the main player in blocking the chemicals that ultimately interfere with BDNF production.

There are two major factors that interfere with normal BDNF production, inflammation and oxidative stress. Thankfully, dietary interventions can take a bite out of both of these negative influences on BDNF. Just make sure you are consuming ample omega-3 fatty acids, particularly

from fish, and a variety of colorful antioxidants, and you will be maximizing your BDNF production throughout life. Sadly, only 18 percent of
North Americans eat fish and shellfish two or more times per week. Try
your best to get into the habit of regular fish consumption, and if you
can't, make sure you supplement with fish oil capsules every day. New
enteric-coated fish oil capsules rich in EPA are available in North
America (o3mega+joy™) and they do not have the typical odor and fishy
repeat of standard fish oil capsules.

The often reported concern that omega-3 supplements are unstable
and may promote free radical damage unless co-administered with vitamin E is in fact an Internet myth. Dr. Trevor Mori and his group from the
University of Western Australia have shown in a number of published
studies that both dietary fish and omega-3 supplements significantly
decrease urinary markers of oxidative stress. In fact, supplements of pure
EPA and DHA reduced urinary excretion of F2-isoprostanes (oxidative
stress marker linked to Alzheimer's disease) by an incredible 27 percent.
The Internet confusion comes from old test-tube studies; the reality in
human beings is that fish oil reduces oxidative stress. What we should be
concerned about is using oils such as high-quality olive oil for deep frying
and not using the same oil in a pan for repetitive cooking, a practice that
promotes oxidative stress and taxes our detoxification system. Once you
see smoke rising from a pan with oil on it, you can be sure that you will
be consuming toxic compounds. Choose canola oil for cooking because it
is more resistant to breaking down at higher heat.

Relationships between higher intake of omega-3 fatty acids (in the
form of fish and seafood) and lower rates of various brain conditions have
been noted. Conversely, the relatively rapid withdrawal of omega-3 and
the introduction of saturated and trans fats as a contributing factor to
mental and cognitive decline have also been noted. Dr Abel Bult-Ito and
colleagues from the University of Alaska have discussed the devastating
effect of rapidly replacing the omega-3-rich traditional diets of northern
polar regions with the Western-style diet. Once these circumpolar communities lose their isolation from Western diet and lifestyles, they have
increased rates of depression, anxiety, suicide, and other mental disorders.
While the researchers acknowledge the importance of cultural and social
issues, the nutritional voids, and omega-3 withdrawal in particular,
emerge as a potentially huge contributor to the decline in mental health.

When you look at the number of brain-related conditions that have been associated with low levels of omega-3 fatty acids and/or where supplemental fish oil appears to be helpful, it is obvious that omega-3s emerge as a dietary superstar for brain health. The range of conditions is enormous, everything from early IQ to late-life Alzheimer's. When researchers see one dietary factor associated with so many neurological and psychiatric conditions, it serves to highlight the importance of these fats, and it is a huge red flag that something must be missing from our modern diet. It may depend on your genetic susceptibility—one man's anxiety in the face of an omega-3 deficiency might be another man's depression or Alzheimer's disease. Without proper fatty acids and nutritional support, one child's violent behavior might be another's attention deficit, low exam scores, or migraines. While there are no guarantees, dietary and supplemental omega-3 fatty acids may be the most significant brain insurance policy you can purchase. I could fill this book with the research connecting omega-3 fatty acids and brain disorders; instead, I will focus on the omega-3 and depression story as a means to highlight the two.

Omega-3 and Depression

There is no question that depression is an extremely complex disorder, one that is influenced by genetics, life stressors, environment, and the individual's brain biology and physiology. Depression can cause significant disability, particularly because it interferes with daily functioning, motivation, and sleep. Up to 20 percent of North Americans experience the symptoms of depression, often severe enough that it can diminish their ability to enjoy life. Over the last hundred years, the overall incidence of depression has increased. The real surge occurred post-1945, and rates today are up to twentyfold higher, with more and more young people experiencing depression at an earlier age. In fact, according to the largest national survey published in the *Archives of General Psychiatry* (2005), all mental health conditions are on the rise. As we begin the twenty-first century, it is now a reality that one in every two Americans will have a diagnosable mental condition at some point in their life. It is certainly tempting to write off the rise in depression as simply a matter of changes in attitudes of health professionals or society, or perhaps changes in diagnostic criteria or reporting. Research, however, indicates that this is not the case, and the rise in depression appears to be related to environmental factors. Nutrition is of course one variable that may be a factor, and it is entirely possible that inadequate omega-3 intake, along with the overconsumption of omega-6, trans, and saturated fats, may influence rates of depression. Interestingly, the surge in depression post-1945 coincides with the mass introduction of omega-6 fatty acids into the food supply in the form of inexpensive vegetable oils.

There are several lines of evidence to support a connection between omega-3 fatty acids and various forms of depression. To start with, a number of studies have shown that both intra-nation and international fish and seafood consumption appears to be protective against depression, seasonal affective disorders, bipolar (manic) depression, and postpartum depression. Dr. Joseph Hibbeln and his colleagues from the National Institutes of Health have paved the way in this area of research. He has consistently shown that nations consuming higher amounts of fish and seafood have lower rates of the aforementioned depressive conditions. Australian and European researchers have also shown that fish consumption within a nation is associated with a lower risk of depression and higher mental health status. As interesting as these studies are, they do not prove that an omega-3 fatty acid deficiency is responsible for depression. As the saying goes in research, correlation does not prove causation. However, to add to the strength of the epidemiological studies, scientists have found that those with depression indeed have lower levels of omega-3 fatty acids in blood, and a 35 percent reduction in fat storage cells. Finding a lower level of omega-3 in fat storage cells (adipose tissue) is reflective of one- to three-year dietary intake. Clearly, patients with depression are not taking in these important nutrients, not absorbing them, and/or not metabolizing them.

EPA appears to be a key player in depression, as the lower the level of this important omega-3 fatty acid, the more severe the depressive state. Further background comes from studies of the consequences of inadequate omega-3 fatty acids in experimental settings. Deficiencies of omega-3 fatty acids in animals can lead to alterations in the levels and functioning of two important neurotransmitters, serotonin and dopamine, both of which are involved in human behavior and mood. The brain changes observed in states of animal omega-3 deficiency are remarkably similar to those

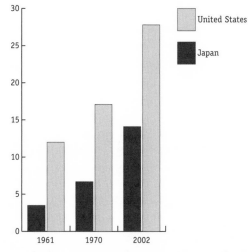

Vegetable oil consumption in kg per person in 1961, 1970, and 2002.

found in autopsy studies of depressed humans. Omega-3 deficiency also decreases normal blood flow to the brain, another interesting finding given the consistent observation that patients with depression have compromised blood flow to a number of brain regions. In addition, an omega-3 deficiency leads to a breakdown in the normal functioning of the blood-brain barrier; this of course allows chemicals that are normally excluded to gain access to the brain. Once inside, these chemicals can damage delicate brain cells and disturb normal communication from cell to cell. Finally, an omega-3 deficiency has been shown to decrease brain phosphatidylserine levels, an important part of the brain cell structure. At least two studies have shown that phosphatidylserine has its own antidepressant activity when supplemented in humans.

The experimental studies have also uncovered mechanisms whereby omega-3 fatty acids might have antidepressant effects. DHA provides structural support to the nerve cell, much like scaffolding, while EPA is responsible for signaling and communications inside and between nerve cells. EPA, as mentioned, may be a key player in maintaining levels of BDNF, the nerve growth chemical that is low in depression. In addition, EPA inhibits the immune chemicals called cytokines, particularly IL-1 beta and TNF alpha, which appear to promote depression and anxiety and impair cognitive function. Inadequate omega-3 allows cholesterol and other fats to take up residence in the nerve cell and it becomes hard and inflexible. The end result is that even in the presence of antidepressant medications, proper neurotransmission from cell to cell is compromised.

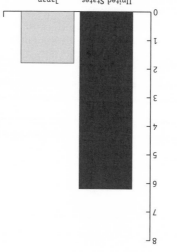

Animal fat consumption in kg per person in 2002.

As effective as some antidepressants and behavioral interventions might be, there is still a large percentage of individuals who are treatment resistant or who do not recover to a satisfactory degree. Consider that the go-to antidepressant medication class of selective serotonin reuptake inhibitors (SSRI) produces a 50 percent improvement of symptoms in only about half of those who maintain therapy, while about 30 percent discontinue therapy before a six-week trial is complete. Obviously, there is room for improvement, and omega-3 fatty acids from fish oil are emerging as an inexpensive means to improve treatment.

As exciting as all the epidemiological and experimental studies are, they serve only to set the stage for clinical studies to determine if indeed omega-3 fatty acids can improve human mood and behavior. The first trial of fish oil with a placebo control took place in 1999 and involved patients with bipolar (manic) depression. This Harvard study, published in the *Archives of General Psychiatry*, showed that very high doses (9.6 g) of EPA and DHA could improve the condition. Specifically, there were longer periods of remission and significant improvements in depressive symptoms. While old dogma suggested that DHA was responsible for the benefits, some researchers suspected that only low levels of pure EPA might be the key. In a study in early 2002, published in the *American Journal of Psychiatry*, researchers found that just 2 g of pure EPA could improve the symptoms of treatment-resistant depression. The investigators found that the EPA, not the placebo, significantly improved depressive symptoms when the oil was added on top of antidepressants that were not working. Results were noted after about three weeks of EPA use, and, very importantly, there were no significant adverse events reported from the pure EPA. In an even larger study, published in the *Archives of General Psychiatry* (2002), researchers were able to look at various doses of pure EPA to determine if one dose was better than another. Interestingly, just 1 g of EPA outperformed a daily dose of 2 g and 4 g, and outperformed the placebo when taken over three months. Once again, the subjects in the study were depressed patients who were unsuccessfully taking antidepressants. The 1 g daily dose of EPA led to significant improvements in depressive symptoms, sleep, anxiety, lassitude, libido, and suicidal thoughts.

In yet another study, this one from Taiwan Medical University, investigators found that a 2:1 ratio of EPA to DHA (4.4 g and 2.2 g respectively) could alleviate depression versus placebo in those with treatment-resistant depression. Once again, the fish oil was well tolerated and no adverse events were reported. As the research intensifies, it is becoming clear that EPA is the main player in mood disorders. Two studies that have examined pure DHA have found that it is no better than placebo in the treatment of depression and postpartum depression. Similar findings have been noted in attention deficit disorders of childhood, where pure DHA has been found to be no better than placebo in two studies, while in three others, which have at least some EPA, the investigators have found beneficial results. I'm not discounting DHA; just make sure your fish oil preparation has some EPA. In pregnancy and lactation, where DHA is critically important, make sure you are getting at least 300 mg of DHA per day.

Outside of major depressive disorder itself, there is some evidence that omega-3 fatty acids can influence depressive symptoms in other conditions. Antarctic krill oil, at doses containing 400 mg EPA and 240 mg DHA, has been shown to improve depressive symptoms associated with premenstrual syndrome. In addition, Harvard researchers found that just 1 g of pure EPA could improve the symptoms of borderline personality disorder. This condition, one that is notoriously difficult to treat, is characterized by both aggression and depression. In this two-month study, the EPA had a mood-regulating effect, improving both depression and aggression over placebo.

Given that omega-3 fatty acids cannot be patented and are outside of the financial juggernaut known as the pharmaceutical industry, it is remarkable that such incredible research has been conducted. University researchers clamor for scarce research dollars when it comes to nutritional interventions; their efforts in this area should be commended. Of course, we have a ways to go before omega-3 fatty acids are routinely recommended for depression. However, the solid research in the area of depres-

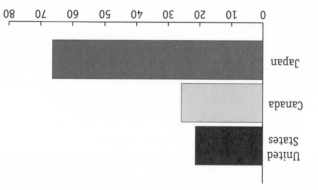

Fish and seafood consumption in kg per person in 2002.

sion is highlighting that the fats we put in our mouths can affect our brain and ultimately our behavior. Dietary omega-3 fatty acids from fish, seafood, plants, and supplements may prevent depression and indeed numerous other brain-related medical conditions.

Omega-3 Sources

The parent omega-3 fatty acid (alpha-linolenic acid) is found in the oils from ground flaxseeds, canola, walnuts, and a range of dark green leafy vegetables. In addition, there are higher levels of alpha-linolenic acid in free-range meats and eggs. Buffalo meat in particular has high levels of the parent omega-3. Hellman's® has a brand new, and great tasting, canola oil–based mayonnaise which is a wonderful way to incorporate the parent omega-3 into the diet with sandwiches and salads. Thankfully, steps are being taken to return omega-3 fatty acids to the modern food supply.

It should be mentioned that alpha-linolenic acid must be converted (in our liver) into heart and brain healthy EPA and DHA. Humans can convert the parent omega-3 into EPA and DHA to only a limited degree, and this conversion is compromised in states of stress, ill health, and when there are even marginal nutritional deficiencies. Folic acid, zinc, and selenium are all involved in the conversion of alpha-linolenic acid into EPA and DHA, and interestingly, low levels of all three of these nutrients have been tied to human depression. The good thing about fish and seafood, and fish oil supplements, is that they already contain the EPA and DHA in preformed state. Along the food chain the algae supplies the parent omega-3 and then fish perform the conversion.

The table below highlights the sources of EPA and DHA in fish and seafood, and the table on the next page shows how our top-heavy omega-6 diet comes from the cooking oils we commonly use in North America.

Stay away from frozen breaded whitefish, because when it comes to increasing your omega-3 fatty acids intake, fish sticks are not the answer. You would need to eat thirty-eight servings of fish sticks each week to get

Various Sources of EPA and DHA	
Fish/Seafood	**Total EPA/DHA (mg/100 g)**
Mackerel	2300
Chinook salmon	1900
Herring	1700
Anchovy	1400
Sardine	1400
Coho salmon	1200
Trout	600
Spiny lobster	500
Halibut	400
Shrimp	300
Catfish	300
Sole	200
Cod	200

to the recommended minimal levels of EPA and DHA. In any case, this type of frozen fish is high in trans or hydrogenated fats, with these bad guys outnumbering the good omega-3s by about 10:1. Researchers from the Medical University of South Carolina have shown that animals fed a high trans fat diet (10 percent) have much more difficulty with simple memory tasks than those fed on non-hydrogenated vegetable oil. Animals in the non–trans fat group performed five times better in straightforward recall tasks. In following with this evidence, researchers from the Rush Institute for Healthy Aging in Chicago found that those consuming the highest amounts of trans fats have a much higher risk of Alzheimer's disease (up to five times higher) than those consuming the least amounts of dietary trans fats.

Dr. Dariush Mozaffarian and colleagues from Harvard Medical School showed just how dangerous eating deep-fried fish can be. Dr. Mozaffarian found that regular consumption of fried fish and fish sandwiches (typical of fast-food joints) increased hardening of the arteries and other cardiac problems. The study, involving more than five thousand older Americans, showed that broiled or baked fish were more likely to have a beneficial effect on signs associated with cardiovascular disease. Clearly then, whitefish, deep-fried on a bun, with low levels of omega-3 and high levels of trans fats and dressed up with soybean oil–based mayonnaise is *not* a means to prevent brain-related conditions . . . such choices may actually be compromising your brain function.

Omega-6 and Omega-3 Content (%) of Dietary Oils		
Oil	Omega-6	Omega-3
Safflower	75	0
Sunflower	65	0
Corn	54	0
Cottonseed	50	0
Sesame	42	0
Peanut	32	0
Soybean	51	7
Canola	20	9
Walnut	52	10
Flax	14	57

What About Contaminants in Fish?

As the research papers pour in, more and more health-care providers and individuals are using fish oil supplements as a means to prevent and treat brain-related conditions, from pregnancy to old age. The question asked by many is "Are fish oil supplements safe?" and the research on contaminants found in fish makes this a valid question. First, let's discuss dietary fish.

The two main contaminants found in dietary fish, mercury and polychlorinated biphenyls (PCBs), have been shown to have a negative impact on human health. San Francisco physician Jane Hightower and her colleague Dan Moore made international headlines when they showed that mercury levels in affluent consumers of fish may be responsible for a host of vague symptoms such as fatigue, headache, decreased memory, decreased concentration, and other cognitive complaints. They measured mercury in the blood of eighty-nine patients with such symptoms and found that high-end fish consumption was associated with mercury in the participants. Swordfish and tuna in particular were significant contributors to mercury elevation. When they pulled the fish out of the patients' diet, the mercury levels declined, and the cognitive symptoms eventually improved.

Other studies have found that even low levels of mercury intake from regularly consumed fish can have negative effects on neuropsychological functioning in otherwise healthy adults. Large predatory fish like swordfish, king mackerel (not to be confused with small Atlantic and Spanish mackerel), shark, and tilefish accumulate significant amounts of mercury, and up to 95 percent is in the highly neurotoxic methyl-mercury form. The mercury in fish is highly bioavailable after human consumption, with close to 100 percent being absorbed from the gastrointestinal tract. The biggest threat is of course to the developing fetus: research shows that consumption of fish high in mercury during pregnancy can cause serious neurological problems. In 2004 Harvard researchers and colleagues from Denmark and Japan reported in the *Journal of Pediatrics* that pre- and postnatal mercury exposure via dietary fish can lead to delays in brain signaling and alterations in the normal variability of the heart rate. The investigators found that mercury exposure in pregnancy resulted in neuropsychological performance deficits in a dose-related manner.

Researchers measured mercury in umbilical cords at birth and hair samples at seven and fourteen years old. Even subtle neurotoxic exposure could have important implications in a child's development and educational achievements. With regard to heart rate variability, it is critically important in adaptation to acute and chronic stress, as well as the prevention of coronary heart disease later in life.

Due to high mercury levels, the U.S. Food and Drug Administration and Health Canada have issued advisories to limit or avoid swordfish, king mackerel, shark, and tilefish during pregnancy. Health Canada recommends fresh and frozen tuna (like tuna steaks and sushi) to be limited to at most one meal per week. Young children, pregnant women, and all women of childbearing age are recommended to restrict tuna intake to once per month. Canned tuna traditionally has been considered low in mercury; however, new FDA data indicates that white albacore tuna has significantly higher levels of mercury than the tilefish that is already on the "do not eat during pregnancy" list. In addition, the FDA research found that bluefish, sea trout, orange roughy, and grouper all have significantly more mercury than tilefish. For more on the FDA mercury testing data, and to help determine individual safe amounts of canned tuna consumption, visit www.ewg.org—this brilliant Web site, home of the Environmental Working Group, even provides a tuna calculator to determine safe limits. Pregnant women should absolutely continue to consume safe fish because the research shows that the greater a woman's low-mercury fish intake during the second trimester, the better the child's mental performance at six months.

The second main concern is related to PCBs, chemical toxins banned in the 1970s because numerous experimental studies connected them with an increased cancer risk. The FDA and the Environmental Protection Agency (EPA) set different standards for safe PCB intake. The FDA levels of 2000 ppb (parts per billion) were set more than twenty years ago and have not been reviewed since that time. In 1999, the EPA set a much lower safe level of PCBs at approximately 10 ppb per week from dietary fish. For now, commercial fish are not subject to these strict EPA guidelines on PCBs. In a large study published in the prestigious journal Science, seven hundred salmon fillets were examined for PCBs. The average level of PCBs in the farmed salmon was 36.7 ppb, and for wild salmon it was only 4.7 ppb. Based on the health risks of PCBs, the

• • • CASE REPORT • • •

Aaron is a nine-year-old boy with attention deficit hyperactivity disorder (ADHD) and bed-wetting (enuresis). His condition was a cause of great concern for his parents, and the bed-wetting in particular was distressing for Aaron. A review of Aaron's diet diary revealed copious amounts of soda, sweets, high-fat snacks, and chocolate. His physical activity was almost nonexistent, with heavy exposure to videogames and television.

The first priority was to clean up the diet and incorporate wholegrain foods to balance out the blood sugar that can soar high and dip low in ADHD. Low-sugar oatmeal and whole-grain cereals became the new substitutes for his previous breakfast, which when it emerged from the toaster was not much more than a block of sugar and artificial flavors/colors. Fiber-containing fresh and frozen fruit, low-fat prepared veggies, and nutritious raw nuts became the only snacks available. Soda was replaced with water and limited amounts of natural juices. Food additives and chemicals were eliminated as much as possible. A children's multivitamin/mineral formula was added, along with 15 mg of zinc and an EPA-rich omega-3 supplement. Contrary to popular belief, pure DHA supplements have not been shown to be of value in ADHD, while studies that used both EPA and DHA have worked well in reducing ADHD symptoms. EPA may be the most important player in the treatment of bed-wetting, and in Aaron's case it made a huge difference.

After one month on the new program, Aaron had mostly dry nights versus the previous month, which had been mostly wet nights. In addition, his behavior and academic performance was reported to be vastly improved. Aaron's commitment to decrease his TV and videogame time and incorporate physical activity into his routine was certainly an important component of his treatment plan. TV and videogames became a reward and a privilege rather than an all-consuming habit.

authors from Cornell University concluded that farmed salmon should be consumed at only one meal or fewer per month. Consumers should note that 90 percent of fresh salmon in North America is farmed salmon, while a large percentage of canned salmon is wild.

It would appear that eating fish and seafood is a little bit scary in today's toxic world. Indeed studies have shown that some of the afore-mentioned research on heavy metals and PCBs in fish has turned away many consumers. That is a real shame, because the research on the ben-efits of fish and seafood consumption from pregnancy to old age is so strong. All it takes is a little effort and application of some cautious prin-ciples when considering fish. Limit the mercury-laden fish, and take advantage of all of the other fish and seafood that are not a concern. Many have been critical of the well-publicized farmed salmon and PCB study because it has turned off so many from salmon without demonstrat-ing a definite cancer risk. A number of experts still suggest that the advantages of farmed salmon, high in omega-3 fatty acids, outweigh any risks resulting from the PCB content. My real concern is not a theoreti-cal human cancer risk associated with PCBs in fish; I'm much more con-cerned about the research surrounding PCBs and mental function. A number of human studies, including one in the *New England Journal of Medicine* (1996) have made clear associations between high-PCB fish consumption in pregnancy and intellectual impairment in the children when assessed years later. In addition, greater intake of high-PCB fish is associated with impairments of memory and learning in older adults, so this is more than a pregnancy concern. Animal studies back up these findings, as they show PCB-induced auditory, visual, memory, and behav-ioral disturbances. Sadly, as researchers pointed out in a study in the *Journal of Urban Health* (2003), low-income families may be more reliant upon locally caught high-PCB fish and seafood.

With all of the media attention on fish contaminants as a back-ground, we can now return to our original question regarding the safety of fish oil supplements. The good news is that oils available today are clean and safe. New molecular distillation techniques allow fish oils to be gently purified so as to not damage them, yet in the process ensure that heavy metals such as mercury, PCBs, and other toxins called dioxins are below detectable limits. Recently, in two separate studies published in *Archives of Pathology and Laboratory Medicine*, Harvard researchers confirmed that commercially available fish oil supplements have less than detectable or only "'negligible amounts" of mercury and PCBs, and organochlorines were not detected at all. In addition to the Harvard research, Consumerlab.com, an independent research group, found no mercury in the twenty fish oil supplements it tested. *Consumer Reports* magazine also tested sixteen supplements in July 2003 and found no significant levels of mercury. Also, a joint investigation from the Canadian national newspaper, the *Globe and Mail*, and Canadian Television (CTV) found that a person would have to take as many as 312 fish oil capsules to be exposed to the amount of PCBs in a single serving of farmed salmon.

The bottom line regarding fish oil supplements? Research from credible groups indicates that supplements available in health food stores, pharmacies, and supermarkets are free of mercury and other contaminants. Writing in the *Archives of Pathology and Laboratory Medicine* (2003), the Harvard researchers state, "due to the lower measured concentrations of mercury in commercial fish oil preparation, consumption of fish oil may be preferable to consuming fish."

Summary

Dietary changes related to fat intake over the last century may be compromising human brain function. The increases in saturated, omega-6 and trans fats, compounded by decreased intakes of omega-3 fatty acids, may have neurobehavioral consequences. Depending on individual experience and genetic susceptibilities, an omega-3 deficiency can present itself in various ways from birth to old age. The administration of omega-3 fatty acids, and the "good" omega-6, gamma-linoleic acid (GLA), has been shown to be helpful in a wide range of brain-related conditions, from improving children's behavior and performance to depression, schizophrenia, multiple sclerosis, and Huntington's disease. In addition to these severe conditions, higher levels of omega-3 intakes are associated with better cognitive function and performance in midlife. On top of this, there are even more studies to indicate that many of today's psychiatric and neurological conditions are associated with low levels of omega-3 fatty acids. Hopefully, in the not too distant future, scientists will unravel these connections and continue to do clinical trials so that we can better understand how omega-3 fatty acids work.

Eicosapentaenoic acid (EPA) is emerging as the brain superstar omega-3. More than encouraging results have been obtained with the administration of pure EPA in depression, chronic fatigue syndrome, schizophrenia, and Huntington's disease. In childhood behavioral disorders and ADHD, studies that have included some EPA in addition to DHA have had successful outcomes. DHA is also critically important; it can be thought of as the scaffolding of the brain and is therefore of extreme importance in fetal development and throughout childhood. Emerging research also suggests that DHA is the main player in maintaining cognitive performance and diminishing the effects of Alzheimer's disease.

Nutritional choices made during pregnancy and early childhood may determine risks of brain-related conditions years later due to effects on genetic expression. Based on international studies, fish and seafood appear to be protective against many neurological and psychiatric illnesses. There is, however, a downside to fish consumption if an individual chooses the wrong kinds of fish. Advisories related to certain fish, including canned tuna, have been issued, with warnings that are directed mostly at women of childbearing age and small children. Adults can also experience subtle and not-so-subtle neurological effects from overconsuming fish high in mercury and PCBs. With just a little effort, you can avoid the fish high in contaminants and take advantage of all the benefits of dietary omega-3 fatty acids. Supplements, including combined EPA/DHA and pure EPA formulas, are available. Fish oil supplements available commercially in North America have been shown to be pure and free of contaminants.

As a final note, it is important to recognize that omega-3 fatty acids should not be viewed in dietary isolation. There are other nutrients that can ultimately influence omega-3 status. Among them, four important dietary factors are also related to brain function—zinc, selenium, folic acid, and overall dietary antioxidants. Zinc (25 mg) has been shown to significantly increase omega-3 status into our cell membranes at the expense of saturated fat. Selenium deficiency can interfere with the conversion of the parent omega-3, alpha-linolenic acid, into brain-healthy EPA and DHA. Selenium deficiency also results in an increase in the omega-6 to omega-3 ratio. Folic acid has been shown to increase omega-3 status when supplemented, and decrease omega-3 status when it is in deficiency in animals. In humans, a diet devoid of antioxidants has been shown to lower blood-essential fatty acids levels, even though there were no changes to dietary fat type or amount. In animals, antioxidants, including ginkgo biloba, have been shown to increase red blood cell levels of EPA at the expense of saturated fat.

This highlights the orchestral nature of human nutrition. Scientifically we have to isolate out nutrients to determine effects, but practically, for those seeking to maximize human brain function and prevent or treat brain-related conditions, omega-3s are but one piece of the nutritional puzzle.

4

Waist Management

HUMANS HAVE BEEN ENJOYING A steady increase in life expectancy over the last thousand years, with a nice boost provided by medical advances and the promotion of public health over the last 150 years. Despite this, there are some red flags being waved—over the last 30 years, North American life expectancy gains have become much smaller, and experts are suggesting that we are headed toward a reversal in the trend. The changes have a lot to do with the type and the amount of food that we put into our bodies, along with the chasers of pollution, lack of intentional physical activity, and stress. This is serious business, and the potential of obesity to shorten the life expectancy of North Americans was brought to the forefront in a well-publicized article in the *New England Journal of Medicine* in 2005. Dr. Jay Olshansky and colleagues from the University of Illinois reviewed the data and, based on our current obesity epidemic, with its obvious connections to diabetes, heart disease, cancer, and other conditions, they see a rapid reversal in gains in health and longevity. Gains that were decades in the making will be undone by obesity and other risk factors associated with our modern lifestyle. In this chapter we will discuss research showing that excess weight, particularly in the abdominal region, is like poison to the brain. In the next chapter, Waste Management, we will see how the buildup of environmental toxins can compromise brain function, setting the stage for a variety of neurological and psychological conditions. While *waist* and *waste* management may seem separate and distinct when it comes to brain health, there is some research suggesting that environmental toxins might promote obesity and interfere with the use of fat as an energy source. More on that in the next chapter, but first let's look at the obesity epidemic and its relationship to brain function.

Obesity is identified by way of the body mass index (BMI), which is the result of dividing weight in kilograms (kg) by height in meters squared (m^2). *Overweight* is defined as a BMI from 25 to 29.9, and *obese* is defined as a BMI of 30 or more. While the BMI certainly has its shortcomings, particularly when it comes to differentiating between lean body mass and body fat, it has been well documented to assist in the evaluation of health risks associated with excess weight. One thing is for sure, the BMI of North Americans was relatively stable until the last thirty years. Through the 1980s and 1990s, massive increases in BMI were noticed in surveys conducted by government health and nutrition examiners. Despite the imperfections of using BMI to determine body fat, it was obvious that the sharp increases were not because we were pumping steel at Muscle Beach in Venice, California. No, the BMI increases were due to carrying excess body fat.

Obesity rates show that in 2000, approximately 65 percent of adults were overweight or obese, and approximately 31 percent were in the obese category. Obesity rates have more than doubled in just thirty short years, and young children growing up today are at much greater risk of being overweight. In the period between 1965 and 2002, the average weight of children between the ages of six and eleven has increased by almost ten pounds! Teens have seen the average weight increase by twelve to fifteen pounds during the same period. On average, both males and females in adulthood are twenty-four pounds heavier today when compared to the mid-1960s. While these are U.S. statistics, the research shows similar trends among Canadians who are now just behind Americans when it comes to weight gain.

So, what does it all really mean when it comes to your brain health? The research is now showing a very strong connection between excess weight and brain dysfunction, both in the neurological and psychological realms. While experts always bring up the connections to diabetes, cardiovascular disease, and cancer, the brain-related consequences seem to fall under the radar. Carrying excess weight has now been shown to be related to depression, anxiety, attention deficit hyperactivity disorder (ADHD), schizophrenia, dementia, Parkinson's disease, and Alzheimer's disease. The fact that being overweight can increase the risk of depression or other psychological conditions seems fairly obvious. Individuals with excess weight score lower on quality of life measurements, have lower self-esteem, and have undoubtedly experienced discrimination in social and economic settings. Children in particular are vulnerable to the stigma of obesity and are less well equipped than most adults to deal with the taunting that goes along with being overweight. For many, being overweight in childhood can be traumatic, setting the stage for depression and related conditions. But what about the reverse situation: could it be possible that depression precedes the development of obesity? Research says yes.

Two separate studies published in the journal *Pediatrics* shows that the odds of becoming obese are dramatically increased later in life if depression is present in early life. Dr. Daniel Pine and colleagues from Columbia University in New York found clear relationships between childhood depression and higher BMI in adulthood when they followed children aged six to seventeen years old for ten to fifteen years. Drs. Elizabeth Goodman and Robert Whitaker from the University of Cincinnati found that the odds of becoming obese doubled in teens who reported a depressed mood at baseline. The risk remained even after the researchers separated out low self-esteem, low levels of physical activity, parental obesity, and lower levels of parent education.

Research also shows that excess weight in midlife predicts higher rates of Parkinson's and dementia, including Alzheimer's. The common thread may be a vicious cycle of high cortisol and abdominal obesity compromising brain health. As research becomes more sophisticated, scientists are beginning to see that it is not so much the body fat per se but rather where it is located that negatively impacts brain functioning. Abdominal fat, or so-called central adiposity (i.e., more fat in the center of your body), is now being recognized as the real threat to human health and brain function. The ratio of waist-to-hip circumference and waist circumference alone have been highly correlated to increased risk of cardiovascular disease, stroke, type 2 diabetes, hypertension, some cancers, and overall premature death. Abdominal fat itself appears capable of biologically affecting mood and cognition and setting the stage for neurodegenerative disease. The chronic and excessive secretion of the stress chemical cortisol may be a major player.

Animal and human studies show that excessive levels of blood cortisol promote insulin resistance and a propensity to gain weight in the abdominal region. One need only look at Cushing's syndrome, where excessive cortisol is the hallmark of the condition. In these patients, there is a significant increase in abdominal fat deposition as measured by advanced CT technology. When patients with high cortisol undergo medical treatment to reduce cortisol, there is generally a significant decrease in intra-abdominal fat stores. In healthy states the enzyme responsible for laying down fat, lipoprotein lipase, is normally kept in check. Lipoprotein lipase has the potential to significantly promote abdominal weight gain because the enzyme activity is two to four times more concentrated within abdominal fat stores versus other areas. Cortisol, it turns out, increases the activity of the lipoprotein lipase, and to make matters worse, the receptors that respond to cortisol in promoting lipoprotein lipase are also two to four times more abundant in abdominal fat versus other areas.

It's definitely a bad situation, but it gets worse. New research published in the journal *Diabetes* by Dr. Ruth Andrew and colleagues from the University of Edinburgh shows that the abdominal fat cells (known as visceral adipose tissue) themselves actually produce cortisol in significant quantities in humans! The fat cells are thus *contributing to the corti*sol production and therefore ensuring that the cycle remains really vicious. Dr. Shigetada Furukawa and his team from Osaka University in Japan have added more fuel to the fire; they have shown that increased oxidative stress within fat cells generates free radicals, which have the potential to do damage throughout the body. Their important paper published in the *Journal of Clinical Investigation* (2004) suggests that obesity induces system-wide oxidative stress, and that oxidative stress inside fat cells causes abnormal secretion of chemical messengers from fat cells. Some of the chemical messengers released from fat cells include tumor necrosis factor-alpha and interleukin-6, both of which can promote inflammation, lower mood, provoke anxiety, and disturb normal cognitive functioning. There was, however, a glimmer of hope from Dr. Furukawa's work—the administration of an antioxidant chemical reduced oxidative stress in the animal portion of the study and helped to regulate, or at least diminish, the dysregulation of chemicals secreted from fat cells. Following this was an eye-opening study presented at the North American Association for the Study of Obesity's Annual Scientific Meeting in Vancouver (2005), where French researchers showed that administration of the important antioxidant Co-enzyme Q10 improved body weight in overweight mice. Innovative drug companies are now working on oral anti-inflammatory and cytokine-lowering medications as a means to combat obesity. Early animal research, some of which was presented at the obesity conference in Vancouver, looks very promising. For now, these studies simply provide more reasons to maximize your dietary antioxidant intake and adhere to the Brain Diet plan.

The idea that obesity promotes body-wide oxidative stress is also supported by a number of studies showing that higher BMI is associated with higher levels of an accurate blood and urine marker of oxidative stress. Researchers have found that the chemical 8-iso-prostaglandin F2, a reliable marker of free radical damage to lipid (fat) components of cells, is associated with inflammation and increased waist circumference. It is interesting to note that this same chemical is elevated in neurodegenerative diseases including multiple sclerosis, Alzheimer's, Parkinson's, and Huntington's diseases. While carrying excess weight earlier in life has not yet been associated with a higher risk of multiple sclerosis, the risk of the latter three conditions may increase with early and midlife obesity. Elevated oxidative stress and inflammatory markers have also been observed in anxiety, attention deficit, depression, and schizophrenia, all of which have been associated with an increased risk of higher BMI and, in most cases, abdominal obesity.

In the last few years, the link between excess weight and the risk of neuropsychiatric conditions has received considerable attention. Dr. Jogin Thakore and colleagues from the Royal London Hospital got the ball rolling in 1997 with a preliminary report showing that patients with major depression have twice the abdominal fat strores of healthy controls. Admittedly, it was a small study, but they did use highly accurate computerized tomography (CT) scanners to determine abdominal fat. They also found a relationship between higher cortisol in the blood and more abdominal fat. Cortisol elevations in depression were clearly associated with an increase in waist circumference. This connection is extremely important because although depression presents in psychologically and physiologically diverse ways, somewhere between 50 and 75 percent of those with depression have elevated cortisol. In a later study (2002), researchers found that it is specifically the depressed patients with high cortisol who have higher abdominal fat. Interestingly, a study published in the journal *Psychiatry Research* (2002) showed that in healthy adults, a larger waist-to-hip ratio was associated with the symptoms of depression and anxiety, and alteration in cortisol production.

Korean researchers underscored the idea that when it comes to fat deposits and depression, location is critical. In an article in *Obesity Research* (2005), they found that specifically abdominal fat is associated with depressive mood in overweight women. German researchers reported in 2005 that abdominal fat deposits were much higher both in depression and in the difficult to treat condition known as borderline personality disorder. The latter condition is characterized by both aggression and depression. They found increased inflammatory cytokines in those with higher abdominal fat, and just in case you forgot, these are the same chemicals that can promote inflammation and compromise cognitive functioning and mood. Also in regard to depression and obesity, a 2005 study by Harvard Medical School researchers showed that a higher BMI is associated with an increased risk of resistance to antidepressant medication.

The obesity and brain connection is not exclusive to depression.

Objective measurements of body fat at middle age are related to a much higher risk of Parkinson's disease later on in life. Dr. Robert Abbott of the University of Virginia and colleagues followed eight thousand healthy males free of Parkinson's disease for thirty years as part of the well-known Honolulu Heart Program. The men were first examined when they were in middle age, at which point various measurements of skin folds were taken. Incredibly, it was discovered that those in the highest skin-fold category had triple the risk of developing Parkinson's disease when evaluated later in life. One of the reasons why researchers ignored the obesity-neurodegenerative disease connection until recently is that advanced clinical presentations of neurological conditions include "wasting" or significant losses of body fat. Such is the case in Huntington's disease, which is considered a disease with characteristic loss of weight in late stages. However, new experimental research in mice in the animal model of Huntington's disease shows that in early life there is actually significant accumulation of body fat and obesity compared to control animals. This connection certainly warrants follow-up in human studies.

Carrying extra weight in midlife is also related to the risk of dementia, according to a well-publicized study in the *British Medical Journal* (2005). The background to the study was more than 10,000 members of the Kaiser Permanente medical care program between the ages of forty and forty-five, who were evaluated for skin-fold thickness and BMI between 1964 and 1973. Fast-forward about thirty years when Dr. Rachel Witmer and colleagues identified who among the 10,276 members (as of 1994) had been diagnosed with dementia. As it turns out, males who were in the highest skin-fold category at middle age had a 72 percent greater risk of dementia, while females had a 60 percent greater risk of dementia. In a separate study published in *Archives of Neurology* (2005), researchers found that in about 1,500 men and women followed for twenty-one years, those with obesity at midlife had double the risk of dementia by the time they reached the ages of sixty-five to seventy-nine.

These results are in line with a study by nutrition and obesity expert Dr. Deborah Gustafson. She and colleagues found that for every 1.0 increase in BMI at age seventy, the subsequent risk of Alzheimer's disease increased by an incredible 36 percent. In the study, they followed healthy subjects for eighteen years and found a clear relationship between baseline weight and subsequent Alzheimer's. They rightly point out that research in this area has been clouded by the fact that in advanced Alzheimer's and even in preclinical states of dementia, a lower BMI is often observed because those with dementia eat less. Incredibly, some researchers had been previously concluding that a low BMI was a risk factor for Alzheimer's disease!

These human studies showing a relationship between obesity and cognitive decline are in agreement with animal studies that show a similar effect. In a study presented at the North American Association for the Study of Obesity's Annual Scientific Meeting in Vancouver (2005), researchers from Tufts University showed that diet-induced obesity alters cognitive performance in rats. Animals fed a diet high in sugar and fat had difficulty with object recognition and were unable to differentiate between novel and familiar objects.

The location of the fat may also be a factor in accelerating the aging process within the brain. In yet another study published in the *Archives of Neurology* (2005), researchers have shown that in men over sixty, the greater the waist circumference relative to hips, the smaller the area of the brain known as the hippocampus. This is the area that governs memory. Incredibly, the inference is that as your waist expands, your cognitive abilities shrink over time.

Psychiatric conditions other than depression have also been associated with abdominal obesity. Using CT technology, researchers have shown that abdominal fat in drug-free patients with schizophrenia is threefold higher than healthy controls. In a separate study, anxiety has also been linked to abdominal fat. Individuals with higher levels of self-reported social anxiety did not differ in actual BMI, however the waist-to-hip ratio was significantly higher. This suggests that it is not body fat itself that is linked to social anxiety, but rather abdominal fat. In addi-tion, a study presented at the North American Association for the Study of Obesity's Annual Scientific Meeting in Vancouver (2005) showed that chronic post-traumatic stress disorder (PTSD) is associated with accumulation of abdominal fat. The researchers from the Veterans Administration Hospital in Virginia suggest that this is likely due to the chronic elevation of stress hormones.

Finally, rates of overweight and obesity have been reported in at least two studies to be much higher in children and adults with attention deficit and hyperactivity disorder versus expected norms. This is surpris-ing, at least in children, where research indicates that ADHD is associ-ated with much higher levels of activity. You would think that they would be less likely to be overweight. It is possible that the condition itself drives patients to overeat sugar and fat-laden foods, and it is also likely that subpar nutritional quality makes a significant contribution to the dis-order itself.

The general theme across neurological and psychiatric conditions is that obesity is bad for your brain. If you are still not convinced, consider Dr. Gustafson's landmark twenty-four-year study that clearly demon-strates the neurotoxicity of obesity. Writing in the journal *Neurology* (2004), the researchers noted that higher BMI over the years was associ-ated with shrinkage of the brain. I'm not joking: Risk of brain atrophy, or shrinkage of brain cells, was 13 to 16 percent higher for every 1.0 increase in BMI. Brain atrophy, well documented to be associated with various neurological and psychiatric conditions, may indeed be provoked by obesity. In the study, those with marked atrophy were on average 1.1 to 1.5 kg/m² higher in BMI (at all examinations) over the years versus those without atrophy.

There is no question that cortisol is emerging as a villain in this obesity-brain relationship. Before ripping it to shreds in a public forum, it is important to recognize that cortisol is a hormone that does some wonderful and amazing things in the human body; at normal concentrations and short-term elevations, cortisol helps us deal with stress, regulates glucose and minerals, maintains arousal and attention, and facilitates memory. When human beings once were threatened by the proverbial saber-toothed tiger, cortisol was worth its weight in gold as it was involved in life preservation. In today's world, however, the saber-toothed tiger is everywhere; it is the forty-five-minute wait to get through the toll booth, the work deadline that rapidly approaches, the noisy neighbor, the angry boss, the person who cuts in front of you, the wait in the doctor's office, the guy reaching for the last Cabbage Patch Doll, and the hordes in a crowded mall, etc. How we perceive these "threats" can make all the difference in the world with regard to your brain health. We will talk about that more in chapter 7, but for now, the point is that cortisol elevations were designed for short-term use only.

After an infrequent stress-related elevation of cortisol, everything goes back to normal in a short time, and balance is once again achieved. That's the world as nature intended. Sadly, chronic stress is extremely common in our world, so cortisol does not get shut down properly. Prolonged elevation of cortisol can lead to cognitive difficulties, fatigue, depression, and a loss of zest for life. When prolonged becomes long-term, elevations in cortisol will lead to shrinkage of brain cells. Yes, the same hormone that contributes to abdominal obesity is the same hormone that attacks nerve cells when in excess. Is it any wonder that abdominal obesity is connected with so many neuropsychiatric conditions?

Cortisol damages nerve cells by a number of mechanisms, including overexciting the neuron by promoting excess NMDA, an "excitatory" neurotransmitter that wreaks havoc when in excess. Cortisol also causes alterations of calcium levels inside the nerve cell and decreases the uptake of glucose, the primary fuel for brain function. This, combined with the free radical damage induced by cortisol, results in a beaten and hapless neuron, a mere shell of its former self. The structural changes, along with the electrophysiological and metabolic dysfunctions, ultimately disturb cognitive function and behavior. Even in states of mild cognitive impairment and in healthy adults, higher cortisol levels predict cognitive deficits. At the extreme end of the cognitive spectrum, higher levels of cortisol have been associated with brain atrophy (shrinkage) in Alzheimer's disease.

While there were some twenty years of experimental studies showing that cortisol promotes brain aging in animals, it was only in 1998 that the first human research was presented. Dr. Sonia Lupien and her colleagues from McGill University, writing in the journal *Nature Neuroscience*, showed that long-term exposure to cortisol promotes the aging process in the hippocampus, an area of the brain responsible for memory and cognition. Indeed, high and rising cortisol levels were related to a 14 percent reduction in the volume of the hippocampus over the course of five years versus those in the lower cortisol bracket. To make matters worse, the hippocampus itself is responsible for turning off or dampening cortisol, thereby setting up a vicious cycle of cortisol elevation.

Cleary, we need to keep additional body fat off and keep our cortisol in check. Dietary fiber may be one means to keep cortisol in check; for example, research shows that a fibrous breakfast cereal consumed in the morning can lower stress and cortisol levels. Unfortunately, fiber is overlooked by most popular weight loss plans. There are countless weight loss books on the market; a few have risen to the top, and the euphoria usually comes and goes. This was clearly evident in 2002, when Americans went no-carb crazy. The science supporting a minimal carb diet for long-term weight loss was paper thin, yet we jumped on a bandwagon driven mostly by testimonials. They gave us lower carbohydrates and the same amount of or even more calories. Thankfully, the high-protein bacon, butter, eggs, steak, chicken, and no-carbohydrate nonsense is fading into the distance as North Americans become aware of the value of fiber, whole grains, and fruits and vegetables. There is no question that dietary fiber can aid in weight management. Higher fiber intake is associated with lower body weight and body fat and emerges as even more important than other nutrients with regard to BMI. Fat and sugar intake cannot be discounted, but low fiber consistently predicts higher body fat content.

Dr. Joanne Slavin of the University of Minnesota uncovered the glaring holes in popular diet plans like Atkins and South Beach. Based on her research, published in the journal *Nutrition* in 2005, the maintenance portions of the daily diet plans provide for only 3 g of fiber a day in South Beach and only 5 g of fiber in Atkins. Given that adults need between 25 and 38 g of fiber per day, depending on age and gender, Dr. Slavin refers to these diets as "woefully inadequate" in fiber. Given the wealth of research on fiber and weight management, I support her position.

Fiber allows you to eat more and weigh less because it displaces calorie-dense foods and makes you feel fuller. In addition, fiber-rich foods, such as whole grains and fruits and vegetables, provide maximum nutritional and antioxidant support. Refined grains, which are of course are basically fiber-free, are stripped of important nutrients. Compared to whole grain wheat flour, white flour contains 41 percent less folate, 41 percent less vitamin B12, 52 percent less selenium, and 75 percent less zinc. All of these nutrients, and the antioxidants found in fiber-based grains, fruits, and vegetables, have been shown to be related to protection of the brain and promotion of normal nervous system functioning. Low levels of all of these nutrients have been linked to depression and lowered mood. In addition, they can influence essential fatty acid and omega-3 levels. So, if you want to keep the weight off, follow the principles of the Brain Diet plan, and add more fiber to your diet.

Eating fish is a good idea also, because omega-3 fatty acids have been shown in two recent studies to enhance weight loss efforts. Researchers from the Institute of Endocrinology in the Czech Republic showed that omega-3 fatty acids added to a low-calorie diet for three weeks (versus placebo) resulted in greater weight loss compared to the low-calorie diet alone. In fact, the omega-3 group had a greater reduction in hip circumference (7.8 cm) than those in the low-calorie plus placebo group (2.5 cm). Not bad, and this follows an Australian study by Dr. Peter Howe which showed that compared to sunflower oil and exercise, fish oil and exercise is the ideal combination for maximum weight loss results. Fish oil supplements seem to turn on enzymes that are involved in the burning of fat during physical activity. These studies support a host of animal studies showing that different fats, despite having the same calorie content, are metabolized differently. Saturated fats—those from butter, cream, milk, ice cream, and meats—are preferentially stored in the abdominal region, and once there they are difficult to mobilize. In contrast, fish, canola, and olive oils are more likely to be stored within lean muscle areas and are more readily mobilized for use as energy.

In one eye-opening study investigating different fats in obesity and diabetes, researchers were surprised to find that despite the same grams of fat per day, and the same calories per day, animals fed soybean oil were 40 percent heavier than a fish oil group. This red flag becomes even more alarming when you consider the U.S. intake of soybean oil has risen from 6.8 kg per person/per year in 1961 to more than 22 kg per person/per year in 2002. But wait, what about in Japan where the rates of overweight and obesity are only one-third that of the United States, don't they eat loads of soybean oil? Actually, they don't come close to Americans. Japanese intake of soybean oil was 1.3 kg per person/year in 1961 and even in 2002 (last available statistics) it was only 5.3 kg. I'm not ready to point the fin-ger at soybean oil alone, but the mass introduction of vegetable oils and the disappearance of omega-3 from the food supply appears to be at least one contributing factor in waistline expansion.

I am often asked about dietary supplements for weight loss, and which ones I recommend. In truth, there is very little in the way of research to support dietary supplements in human weight loss. There are, however, a few exceptions, and with all of the collateral brain benefits associated with fish oil and green tea supplements, those seeking to lose weight should give them consideration. In addition to the fish oil described above, an emerging star in weight loss is green tea, or more specifically the epigallocatechin-gallate (EGCG) that is in green tea. A host of ani-mal studies are now backed up by encouraging human research showing that green tea can enhance the burning of fat as energy and the reduction of abdominal fat. Human research, published in the *American Journal of Clinical Nutrition* (1999), showed that 270 mg of EGCG can increase daily energy expenditure without affecting heart rate or inducing side effects. Green tea appears to open up doors in fat cells that are associated with the use of fat as energy, yet it does not affect overall food intake. A second human study, published in the journal *Phytomedicine* (2002), showed that 270 mg of EGCG daily was able to decrease body weight by 4.6 percent and waist circumference by 4.5 percent when taken for twelve weeks by moderately obese patients.

In January 2005, an eye-opening study was published in the *American Journal of Clinical Nutrition*; Japanese researchers led by Dr. Tomonori

Nagao showed that 690 mg of green tea catechins (136 mg EGCG) per day for twelve weeks led to significant reductions in waist circumference, BMI, body fat, and body weight. Most notable was the incredible twenty-seven-square-centimeter reduction in abdominal fat versus placebo. It is also important to note that this was a well-designed study that used CT scan technology to verify this reduction in abdominal fat. Also, in July 2005, researchers writing in the journal *Obesity Research* showed that green tea (270 mg EGCG daily) and moderate caffeine (150 mg) improved the maintenance of weight loss.

In addition to these studies, I was also involved in a research project, led by University of Toronto veteran researcher Dr. Venket Rao and Toronto physician Dr. Kathee Andrews, which investigated the value of a commercial weight loss formula called abs+™. In this study, three months of abs+™, providing a dose of 270 mg EGCG, led to significantly more body weight loss than placebo. In the abs+™ group, the majority lost weight versus those in the placebo group where most gained weight. Once again, there were no significant adverse events reported.

Next, if you are actively seeking to lose weight, consider a meal replacement. Government-approved meal replacements (not protein shakes) are supported by a wealth of research and emerge as the most important dietary supplement when it comes to human weight loss. In the *International Journal of Obesity* (2003), researchers pooled all the data on meal replacements up to January 2001. They concluded that meal replacements safely and effectively produce significant weight loss and decrease risk factors associated with weight-related disease. From 2001 to 2005, the research has continued to validate meal replacements as effective weight loss supplements. In fact, convenience and compliance are rated higher in meal replacement groups than low-fat, calorie-controlled diets alone. The challenge for health-conscious consumers is finding a meal replacement that meets government requirements for a meal replacement and yet is free of sugar and food dyes common to many products. Thankfully, healthy versions of meal replacements such as nutrilean+™, which doesn't contain sugar and includes of more fiber and antioxidants, are emerging from the nutritional supplement industry (see the Appendix). A healthy meal replacement drink (or food bar) fixes portion size and eliminates the need to be concerned with counting calories for at least one meal. This is important because in today's super-sized world, portion sizes, and ultimately calories, are misjudged by 33 to 200 percent, i.e., consumers think they are actually consuming far fewer calories than they really are.

In relation to the brain diet, it is interesting to note that calorie restriction, without malnutrition, has been shown to extend lifespan in a variety of species, from yeast to fruit flies, from mice to monkeys. The experimental studies on calorie restriction do not involve starvation because there is maintenance of essential nutrients. The calorie restriction studies are in essence the opposite of what is happening in today's obesity-prone society, where we have loads of calories and minimal nutrient intake. Think about it: the very foods that can make us fat—soft drinks, sweets, cakes, ice cream, etc.—are the foods with minimal to no nutritional value. Not only does calorie restriction consistently extend the length of life, it also lowers biomarkers associated with brain aging, such as increased oxidative stress. In animal models of both Parkinson's disease and Alzheimer's disease, calorie restriction has been shown to prevent the normal course of brain decline.

Research by Dr. Mark Mattson of Johns Hopkins University shows that intermittent—every other day—fasting is beneficial for health, brain function, and longevity in animals. When meal size and frequency are reduced in rodents, they are less likely to succumb to environmental toxins and extreme stressors. Interestingly, intermittent fasting is associated with enhanced learning and memory, as well as decreased activity of the sympathetic nervous system (stress branch) and better adaptation to stress. On the other hand, overeating is associated with increased sympathetic tone and a lower adaptation to stress. Also, intermittent fasting can increase levels of our old friend BDNF, the brain chemical responsible for maintaining the integrity of the nerve cells throughout life.

The potential benefits of intermittent fasting and caloric restrictions are enormous, but researchers are a long way from establishing a proven protocol for humans. The message here is not to drastically cut calories in an effort to prevent or treat neurodegenerative disease. The benefits of calorie restriction should be interpreted as just one more reason to follow the Brain Diet, say "Minimize It!" (vs. super-sizing), and use portion control to maintain a healthy weight.

Calcium is also an emerging story in weight loss. A lack of dietary calcium leads to enhanced storage of fat and a reduction in the breakdown

of fat as energy. It is as if low calcium tells the body that there is a nutritional emergency and it's time to conserve. There is now significant
research indicating that lower intakes of dietary calcium are associated
with a greater risk of obesity in adults and children. According to research
in the *Journal of the American College of Nutrition* (2002), the percentage
of young women aged nineteen to twenty-six with average calcium intake
(500 mg day) who are overweight is around 17 percent. That number
drops significantly to 3.6 percent in women who take in 1100 mg a day.
Based on the research, an average adult taking in only 300 mg of calcium
is projected to weigh eighteen pounds more than an adult (same age and
gender) taking in 1300 mg of calcium per day. Also, although advertising
would have you believe that only dairy calcium can give you the weight
loss benefits of calcium, researchers from the University of Colorado
found otherwise. Writing in the *International Journal of Obesity* (2003),
these investigators found that total dietary calcium, and not only dairy-
based calcium, increased fat burning over twenty-four hours.

Dietary and supplemental calcium is an extremely important part of
the Brain Diet, not only because it may help you keep pounds off, but also
because it promotes bone health. Beyond calcium, there are other dietary
considerations in bone health such as plant-based antioxidants. Dr.
Leticia Rao of the University of Toronto has shown that free radicals
interfere with the maintenance of bone mineralization, and that antioxidants can help promote the activity of osteoblasts, the cells that help
form bone. Consider that patients with neuropsychiatric conditions like
Alzheimer's disease and depression have lowered bone mineral density.
Researchers are not exactly sure why, but oxidative stress and cortisol elevations may be common threads.

In addition, alkaline foods, such as fruits and vegetables, help keep
calcium in the bone where it belongs. Western diets are notoriously top-
heavy in acidic meats and grains and low in alkaline fruits and vegetables.
The human blood must be kept at a critical pH, very close to neutral; any
deviation can lead to death. Given that, a diet consistently high in acidic
foods will leach calcium out of the bones in order to maintain blood pH
because to your body, obviously, staying alive in the here and now is a priority over brittle bones later in life. While some have disputed this
acid/alkaline diet connection, a landmark study by Swiss researchers in
the *American Journal of Physiology—Renal Physiology* (2003) showed that

the Western diet is associated with a mild acid excess and elevation of cortisol. In turn, the cortisol elevations are associated with increased risk of fracture. An alkaline diet neutralized the effects of the Western diet, reduced cortisol, and improved markers of bone integrity. The implications are that not only does our acid-heavy diet devoid of fruits and vegetables promote osteoporosis, it also may promote obesity and brain-related conditions by way of cortisol elevations. So, here's yet another reason to increase your intake of a variety of fruits and vegetables, a way to lower cortisol and keep your bones and your brain healthy.

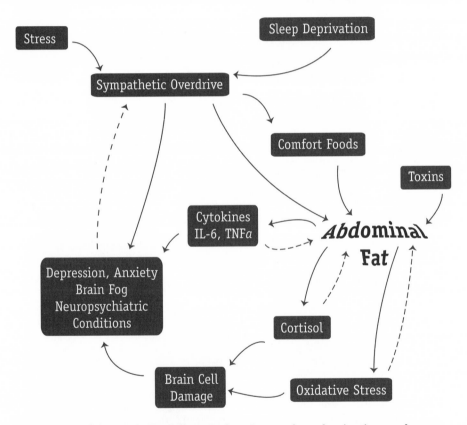

The Most Vicious of all Vicious Cycles: Stress, sleep deprivation, and many brain-related conditions feed the sympathetic (stress) branch of the nervous system. Sympathetic overdrive promotes brain-related conditions and abdominal adipose (fat) deposition. Abdominal fat then adds to the burden of cortisol, oxidative stress, and mood-altering cytokines (immune chemicals). All of these agents and environmental toxins continue to encourage the maintenance of abdominal fat.

It is also important to note that an acid-heavy diet devoid of fruits and vegetables can promote the absorption of the brain-toxic heavy metal aluminum. While it has been a matter of debate for some years, connections can be made between Alzheimer's disease and aluminum accumulation in the brain. What is not debatable at this point is that Alzheimer's patients actually absorb dietary aluminum much more readily than healthy controls. Interestingly, chronic fatigue syndrome patients seem also to absorb more aluminum, as levels in the blood have been reported to be much higher than in healthy adults. Aluminum is well known to interfere with cognitive function. An alkaline diet promotes the elimination of aluminum from the intestinal tract, while an acidic diet actually promotes absorption.

Additional Weight Loss Tips

When it comes to weight loss, most diet plans and books are a bust because they are focused only on the macronutrient. In other words they are low fat, low carb, high protein, or high protein and fat. Not enough emphasis has been placed on fiber and micronutrients like calcium, or spices that have been shown to increase fullness and reduce calorie intake. The same spices that are potent antioxidants and protect nerve cells are also beneficial in weight loss efforts. The popular diet plans have ignored green tea and other polyphenols that may influence long-term fat burning. Also, there has been very little discussion on the research showing that different fats have different effects on the deposition and removal of body fat. The real problem, however, with popular diet plans is that human beings easily tire of eating only chicken, bacon, and eggs, or unpalatable fat-free meals. They fizzle out. Humans need sensible and flavorful meals because, ultimately, long-term weight loss is about compliance. Research clearly shows that better adherence leads to greater weight loss. It follows then, that if a diet plan is not highly restrictive of one food group, then enjoyment will increase, and an individual will stick with the diet. That said, here are some more weight loss tips.

- Give up high-calorie soft drinks; they have been associated with weight gain and oxidative stress. They supply massive calories and little to no nutritional value, and when taken at meal time they may inhibit the normal gut-brain communication that signals fullness in the brain. Don't rely on diet soft drinks as an alternative. Research from the University of Texas has shown that diet soft drink consumption is related to later weight gain in more than one thousand adults followed for over twenty-five years. This follows Purdue University research showing that animals fed the equivalent of diet soda subsequently consume more overall calories versus those consuming a high-sugar sweetener. Cola, both regular and diet, has been linked to high blood pressure.

- Eat at regular times. Those who eat at irregular times eat about 100 more calories per day.
- Eat breakfast. Those who skip breakfast have consistently been shown to eat more calories through the day.
- Drink adequate amounts of water.
- Eat slowly.
- Follow the advice in the Dietary Context chapter.

In closing, the ultimate weight management diet plan was uncovered in 2003 by Dr. P. Kirstin Newby and her colleagues from the U.S. National Institutes of Health. Writing in the *American Journal of Clinical Nutrition* (2004), they report that the diet with the highest success rate in preventing increases in BMI and waist circumference is one high in fruits, vegetables, reduced-fat dairy, and whole grains and low in red and processed meat, fast food, and soft drinks. So the secret is out: if you want to keep your weight in check, this is the diet of choice.

Summary

Obesity, particularly among children, is now a global epidemic. More than one billion people worldwide are now overweight, a figure expected to rise to one and a half billion in less than ten years. As the research evolves, it is becoming clear that abdominal fat is the real villain when it comes to brain dysfunction. Excess body weight and abdominal fat in particular have been associated with numerous neurological and psychiatric conditions. Carrying excess weight has been shown to predict later onset of depression, Alzheimer's and Parkinson's disease. Excess abdominal fat has been associated with depression, schizophrenia, and anxiety disorders. The stress hormone cortisol may be playing an important role in establishing and maintaining abdominal fat. Cortisol is secreted from fat cells into circulation and has the potential to damage the brain and promote further abdominal weight gain. Fat cells also generate free radicals, which can damage tissue located far beyond the original fat cell. In addition, fat cells secrete immune chemicals called cytokines which promote further free radical damage and inflammation.

The good news is that weight loss can help cut off this vicious cycle. Don't look to fad diets to promote long-term weight loss results—instead, follow the dietary pattern scientists from the National Institutes of Health found to be most protective against an increase in BMI and waist circumference. It is very straightforward: eat plentiful fruits, vegetables, whole grains, reduced-fat dairy, and limit your consumption of red and processed meats, fast food, and soft drinks.

When it comes to the sea of weight-loss supplements, most are useless. There are some credible exceptions. Fish oil, green tea, calcium, and meal replacement drinks and bars may be worth considering. These, however, are supplements, and not substitutes for the healthy diet pattern shown to keep the weight off. Finally, when it comes to weight management, the actual food you eat is, of course, central to any plan; however, the concept of dietary context is often overlooked by the popular diet books. Dietary context considers non-nutritional lifestyle factors that play a huge role in weight management. This area includes stress management, mind-body medicine, exercise, sleep, and other lifestyle influences that have an impact on weight management and brain health. We will take that up in chapter 7, but first let's look at toxins and the influence of a healthy gastrointestinal tract on brain function.

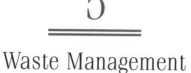

5

Waste Management

W HEN IT COMES TO EXPOSURE to environmental toxins, research shows that the brain is the most sensitive of organs. Even minute amounts of some of the seventy-five thousand chemicals in commercial use in North America can cause neurobehavioral changes. Remember when we talked about how exciting it is that nutrition can influence genetics? Well, thanks to a growing body of research, the influence of *toxins* on genetics is also becoming apparent. When it comes to how you think and behave, the shaping of your personality traits, and your risk of brain-related conditions, genetics do play an important role—but it is how the genes are influenced by the environment that is critically important. The influence of environmental chemicals on human brains can range from subtle cognitive difficulties to more severe mood alterations, or even major neurodegenerative diseases. Even chemicals that are now banned, such as certain organochlorine pesticides, are still wreaking havoc in humans some thirty years later.

As stated by Dr. Kaye Kilburn in the journal *Archives of Environmental Health* (2003), "It is strange that few psychiatrists, when evaluating chemically exposed patients, consider that depression, mania, and other disorders they treat with drugs (chemicals) could be caused by other chemicals."

Below are just some examples of the environmental chemical load humans have to deal with on a regular basis.

Exhaust fumes	Cigarette smoke	Pesticides	Plastics
Dioxins	Mold	Solvents	Paints
Herbicides	Cleaning supplies	Medications	PCBs
Heavy metals	Cosmetics	Dry cleaning chemicals	
Carpet fumes	Furniture fumes	Preservatives	
Food dyes	Overcooked meats	Synthetic materials	

It takes years of bureaucratic work to get a chemical banned, yet in the interest of profits some two thousand new synthetic chemicals are registered by the U.S. government each year. Environmental toxins are everywhere, and research clearly shows that excessive accumulation of toxins in human tissue is a reality. Incredibly, environmental toxin buildup has been noted even at high elevations in the Canadian Rocky Mountains, clearly indicating that toxins can readily travel via the air. The widespread use of herbicides and pesticides in rural areas is believed to be responsible for the high rates of Parkinson's disease among rural dwellers. Consider also that of the 2.5 million tons of pesticides used worldwide each year, less than 0.1 percent actually reaches the pest. The rest enters your environment, my environment, and that of our neighbors. The chemicals are clearly capable of traveling far and wide, and they persist for years.

Food additives such as monosodium glutamate (MSG) have been linked with increased oxidative stress, worsening of the brain-related symptoms in fibromyalgia, and the induction of anxiety. Aspartame has been shown to provoke symptoms of fibromyalgia, induce seizures and panic attacks, lower serotonin, and diminish memory and cognition. While most appear to tolerate these chemicals, there are numerous reports of children and adults who are sensitive to the effects. An inappropriate leaking of the blood-brain barrier may be a factor for some sensitive individuals.

Artificial food colorings have also been shown to affect the human brain and in particular aggravate the symptoms of hyperactivity in children. In the largest review of the topic, researchers from Columbia and Harvard Universities concluded that food chemicals can be neurotoxic and affect behavior. In their review of fifteen studies, published in the

Journal of Developmental and Behavioral Pediatrics (2004), the consensus was that artificial food colorings can provoke symptoms among many young children with hyperactivity. Following this review was another original double-blind, placebo-controlled study by researchers from Southampton General Hospital in the United Kingdom. They showed that among 277 three-year-olds there were significant reductions in hyperactive behaviors when food additives were withdrawn. In addition, upon challenge with the food colors and a common preservative called benzoate, parents reported much higher levels of hyperactivity in their children versus placebo.

Similar findings have been shown in cases of chronic fatigue syndrome and fibromyalgia where food dyes, preservatives, and other dietary chemicals appear to provoke symptoms. Studies in these two related illnesses have shown significant improvement among patients when various additives and chemicals are removed. The bottom line here is that it is no longer a debate about whether or not food dyes, flavor enhancers, preservatives, and the like *can* affect human brain function or not—the individual effects may come down to genetics, the nature of the particular illness and environmental factors.

Still unknown is the effect of a combination of chemicals that can show up in numerous foods. Quite often the "safety" of chemicals is based only on that single and particular additive. Companies are not forced to, and therefore do not evaluate mixtures of food dyes and preservatives. Research, however, does show a combined effect of artificial food colors and flavoring. Research also shows that other environmental factors such as viruses can enhance the brain-toxic effects of chemicals like MSG.

Let's have a closer look first at pesticides because their consumption with food is, of course, a dietary concern. Since the mid-twentieth century, overall pesticide use has risen by over 3,000 percent, yet amazingly, the overall crop loss to insects has risen by 20 percent in the same time frame. Pesticides find their way into our water and food supplies, and ultimately into our bodies. Of major concern are the various studies that have found significant levels of chlorinated pesticide residues in human breast milk. Research from various geographic localities in the United States and Canada has shown not just one but a variety of environmental chemicals in breast milk, levels of which were highly correlated to the amount of toxins stored in the mother's adipose (fat) cells.

There are a couple of issues here, the most important being the influence of pesticides on delicate pre- and postnatal brain development. However, finding numerous pesticides also brings up the concept of synergy. Remember our discussion about the beauty of dietary antioxidants working together, where the two together have a greater effect than the sum of the individual parts? Well, it appears that environmental pesticides can do the same thing—only in the opposite health direction. Dr. Mohamed Abou-Donia and colleagues from Duke University showed that combinations of pesticides increase behavioral alteration, sensory disturbances, and oxidative stress, and together they are more likely to open up the blood-brain barrier. Like a couple of small-time crooks joining to pull off a big heist, toxic chemicals act together to gain access through the high-security fence around the brain.

In our profit-driven world, if something is safe for a few days, or even a month, it is given the green light for all of us and long-term safety issues are basically non-issues. Peddlers of synthetic chemicals do not have to evaluate short-term safety (forget about long-term safety—it is unknown) in the context of other chemicals, they merely have to provide data on that individual chemical. We have no definite picture of what the combined exposure to environmental chemicals might be doing to our own brain health and that of our children. Clearly, Dr. Abou-Donia's research on the combination of chemicals is alarming, and really, it is a microcosm of how big business works.

Let's focus on pesticides in our environment and the primary reason for being concerned about them in the context of the Brain Diet—neurological and psychological alterations. Overt pesticide poisoning can obviously lead to mental retardation and brain damage, but what about more subtle, low-level exposures, known medically as "sub-clinical doses"? Even low levels can cause oxidative stress, behavioral abnormalities, anxiety, depression, irritability, cognitive difficulties, and fatigue in animal studies. Yes, animals are capable of displaying behaviors reflective of human anxiety and depression. Early pesticide exposure has been shown to induce B vitamin deficiency and alter serotonin function later in life in mammals. Dr. Justin Aldridge and colleagues, again from Duke University (which appears to be the epicenter of environmental toxin research), showed that one of the most heavily used pesticides in the world, chlorpyrifos, has long-term effects after pre- and postnatal exposure. Specifically, they showed that this chemical alters the serotonin function of animals later in life after exposure early in life. The implications are enormous and support other research studies indicating that environmental toxins have long-term effects on serotonin function. Remember that dysfunction of the serotonin system is associated with many brain-related conditions, including anxiety and depression. Dr. Aldridge's work shows that environmental toxins disturb the programmed development of serotonin structure and function, which might add to other risk factors for psychiatric and neurological conditions.

One area where serotonin disturbances may play a significant role is in obesity. It has been known for about thirty years that serotonin is involved in appetite and in satiety. Proper functioning of serotonin at the receptors in nerve cells is required for satiety, both during and after meals. Some serotonin-based drugs were highly effective in weight loss (remember Fen-Phen) but had to be pulled due to side effects. In addition to altering serotonin, environmental toxins may also interfere with actual weight-loss attempts by slowing down metabolism. Dr. Angelo Tremblay and colleagues from Laval University in Canada made headlines when they showed that stored environmental toxins released from fat cells upon weight loss can dramatically turn down the dial on thermogenesis, our ability to use fat as an energy source. Environmental toxins, particularly organochlorines (organochlorine pesticides and industrial polychlorinated biphenyls [PCBs] and dioxins), interfere with the functioning of the mitochondria (the cellular site of energy production), lower the active thyroid hormone (T3), and decrease overall metabolic rate. Writing in the *International Journal of Obesity* (2004), Dr. Tremblay showed that once again it's one of those vicious cycles—those who are overweight have much higher levels of environmental toxin storage (in fat cells), and when released with weight loss they interfere with the breakdown of fat and encourage weight gain. So, the concepts of *waist* and *waste* management are really not that far apart.

Development of the young brain is extremely complex, with countless brain cells dividing, maturing, migrating, making connections with other cells, and establishing their special jobs (differentiation). Think of it like the most finely tuned orchestra in the world, where just one note off key can throw off everyone. Environmental toxins can be that off-key note, disturbing the brain orchestra and leading to impaired learning, altered behavior, IQ deficits, and mood alterations.

Over the last decade, the idea that pesticides can influence the development of serious neurological conditions such as Parkinson's disease has moved from mere suspicion to beyond a reasonable doubt. The research movement is now focused on figuring out which pesticides in particular are the worst offenders. A host of studies have shown that consistent exposure to pesticides leads to cognitive impairments, which may ultimately predict later onset of dementia and other neuropsychiatric conditions. In a study published in the *American Journal of Epidemiology* (2003), Dr. Isabella Baldi and colleagues found that occupational exposure to pesticides was related to lower cognitive performance; they also showed that those occupationally exposed had a 5.6 times greater risk of Parkinson's disease and a 2.4 times greater risk of Alzheimer's disease. In the well-publicized Geoparkinson study, Dr. Anthony Seaton of the University of Aberdeen found that among three thousand people living in five European countries, pesticide exposure was a significant risk factor. Risk increased in a linear fashion, with amateur garden buffs being 9 percent more likely to develop Parkinson's and professional farmers 43 percent more likely to develop the disease. In addition, research in the journal *Toxicological Sciences* (2003) shows that chronic low-dose organophosphate pesticides are also associated with anxiety and depression among agricultural workers. This may explain why in some states farmers have higher rates of major depression and suicide.

Another area of environmental concern is indoor air quality, particularly from what are called volatile organic compounds. These chemicals from building materials, furniture, carpet, paint, cleaning supplies, and plastics are found in significant quantities in indoor air, about ten times that of outdoor levels. Individuals complaining of neurological and psychiatric symptoms as a result of volatile organic chemicals have generally been ignored by the medical community. Symptoms such as headache, brain fog, dizziness, and lack of mental acuity are common complaints of what has now been termed "sick building syndrome."

In a strange twist, it was the EPA building in Washington, D.C., that became the most famous sick building and opened the eyes of doubters. When the EPA completed its new headquarters building in 1988, employees were delighted to move into the new digs. The excitement began to diminish when employees experienced a variety of symptoms—and not just one or two workers; almost one hundred were convinced that the building was making them sick. The issue was pretty much dismissed, so the employees walked out and picketed. Imagine, the EPA's own employees refusing to go into their own building because it was making them sick. The administration stepped up its investigation and indeed uncovered a potential problem. The new carpet was suspected of releasing volatile organic compounds, many of which are known neurotoxins. In the end, the EPA ripped out some twenty-seven thousand square feet of carpet, after which most employees returned to their desks. I wouldn't wish sick building syndrome symptoms on anyone, but I wonder: if the EPA building episode and the subsequent lawsuits had not happened, would the awareness of the issue be at the level it is today? As I am writing this book, there are 500 scientific references to sick building syndrome and 512 references to multiple chemical sensitivity (a related condition) on the scientific database Medline. Prior to 1989, there were no references to multiple chemical sensitivity and only six references to sick building syndrome.

Indoor and "in automobile" black mold exposure can also lead to a host of neurological symptoms, including dizziness, impaired memory, and lack of concentration. Dr. Kaye Kilburn of the University of Southern California is one of North America's leading experts on environmental toxins and subsequent brain impairment. Writing in the *Archives of Environmental Health* (2003), Dr. Kilburn reported that in those with known exposure to household mold, usually the black mold *Stachybotrys atra*, twelve of fourteen brain-related physiological functions were adversely affected. In addition, those exposed to mold have reduced vigor and increased tension, depression, anger, fatigue, and confusion. These results are in line with those found by Dr. Wayne Gordon and colleagues from Mount Sinai School of Medicine in New York. They found that the impact of mold exposure on brain function is not all that different from moderate traumatic brain injury. Let me be clear: the study subjects with mold exposure had *no prior psychiatric history* and there was no evidence of malingering or symptom exaggeration. They were regular folks whose brain functioning changed when they were exposed to mold.

Researchers at Mount Sinai School of Medicine have also shown that adult volunteers have an average of 91 industrial compounds, pollutants, and chemicals in both urine and blood. Of the 167 chemicals identified in this group, 94 are known to be toxic to the brain and nervous system. It is important to point out that none of the individuals tested had an occupation where cleaning with chemicals was a necessity, nor did they live near an industrial facility.

We talked previously, in chapter 3, about the concerns related to mercury contamination in fish and seafood. Mercury and other toxic heavy metals like lead are also present in our environment, and humans can accumulate these toxins in high levels. Some have raised huge red flags about the fact that the dental amalgam (silver filling) is about 50 percent mercury. Many dentists are now switching over to white composites, not only for the health of patients, but also for themselves and those in the dental practice. Consider a recent study in the *International Dental Journal* (2003), where researchers found that dental practice employees have higher blood and urine mercury levels than healthy controls. Not only that, the higher the urinary mercury, the lower the scores on logical memory and memory retention. Psychiatric symptoms were also correlated with urinary mercury, higher levels predicted increased scores on anxiety and psychoticism scales.

Incredibly, some try and defend toxins and dismiss any evidence that low levels may do the brain harm. The general defense is the same one the tobacco companies formerly used—there are thousands of people who have smoked cigarettes for years, some to old age, without developing lung cancer. Holes in that argument were punctured over half a century ago, yet it was only recently that cigarette smoking in public venues finally became regulated. Thankfully there is a small minority of scientists who won't sell out to the big profiteers; they actually care about the "little guy," the medical minority. They are well aware of the fact that millions of people can live to old age in the presence of low levels of environmental toxins, yet they are unwilling to dismiss the plight of those whose lives have been turned upside down by chemical exposure. They are also willing to accept and investigate the reality that environmental toxins can have subtle, and not so subtle, effects on human brain performance and the individual's mood state.

Patients with Alzheimer's and chronic fatigue syndrome have been shown to have higher blood levels of aluminum, and although exposure appears to be no different from healthy controls, the absorption of aluminum may be the critical issue. Doctors from the Jos University Teaching Hospital in Africa showed that blood levels of cadmium and lead were significantly higher in patients with depression and schizophrenia, and zinc levels were lower in both groups. I could fill up this entire book with a discussion of how environmental toxins have the potential to influence the present and future brain health both of you and your children. It really isn't necessary; others such as Dr. Kaye Kilburn have already done an excellent job with that task. The focus here is on protecting yourself and your children against environmental toxins.

Detoxification

We are fortunate that the human body, including the brain itself, is equipped with a brilliant detoxification system. Optimal functioning of the detoxification system is completely reliant upon a variety of important nutrients. Your ability to detoxify is only as good as the quality of your diet. Soft drinks, fast food, preserved meats, cakes, cookies, ice cream, barbequed meats, and the like do very little to help you detoxify.

Within the realm of my discipline, nutritional medicine, "detox" is such a vague term. It gets clouded out by magazine articles and Internet sites where it seems that everyone and their proverbial uncle has the "best" detox plan. The purported "best" can range from complete fasting to special juices and modified diets, or those that involve the taking of many harsh botanical (herbal) ingredients that are very, very upsetting to the gastrointestinal tract.

In order to maximize detoxification, we must maximize our intake of the nutrients and foods that support the body's main detox organs—the liver and the intestines. A healthy and strong gastrointestinal (GI) tract will prevent many toxins from ever gaining access inside the human body. Think of the gastrointestinal system as an extension of the outside skin, acting as the ultimate dividing line between out, and inside. In addition to the intestinal cells, which act as a physical barrier, there are also GI cells, which separate the good from the bad. Like a professional garage sale browser who separates the valuable from the junk in someone's garbage, the GI cells must decide what nutrients to keep in and what toxins to keep out. And unlike garage sale hunters, who only work on weekends, GI cells never get a day off. While things usually work out well, problems arise when stress levels get high and nutritional quality gets low. Both of these factors can make the intestinal wall more permeable to compounds that would normally be excluded. It is yet another vicious cycle—low levels of various nutrients may enhance the accumulation of toxins, and compromise our ability to get rid of them.

The relationship between the GI tract and the brain in both health and disease is critically important and warrants a full discussion in the next chapter. For now, consider that dietary factors that support a healthy GI tract, especially fiber, promote detoxification. Remember that fiber, such as rice or wheat bran, can bind up toxic chemicals for removal from the GI tract. Fiber also promotes the growth of beneficial bacteria within the GI tract. Probiotics, generally defined as live, viable bacteria, can improve health by improving the intestinal microbe balance and can actually lower the levels of potentially toxic chemicals inside the GI tract. In addition, these bacteria protect the intestinal lining to prevent toxins from being absorbed inappropriately. Consider a 2001 study by researchers from Ghent University in Belgium, which showed that the probiotic fermented milk drinks Actimel (by Danone) and Yakult (by Yakult USA) can bind up herbicides and make them less bioavailable. Both of these drinks contain specific strains of the beneficial bacteria *Lactobacillus casei*. Interestingly, the bacteria were necessary for the detox effect, as the milk alone (nonfermented) did not decrease the amount of toxins present. The good news is that both the Actimel and Yakult drinks are available in North America and regular consumption of both should be considered a part of daily detoxification.

You will note that I purposely used the term "daily detoxification." This is because it is much more appropriate to consider detoxification a continuous concept. While many of the so-called "best" plans last from a few days to a week, in today's toxic environment we require constant and steady nutritional support at the liver and GI tract. Protein and phytonutrients from plants are extremely important for liver detoxification. Once chemicals gain access to the human body, the liver becomes Grand Central Station in the effort to remove the toxins. In order to understand how nutrition can influence liver detoxification, it is first helpful to take a closer look at how the liver handles toxins. When a toxin arrives at the liver, it meets up with detoxification enzymes otherwise known as biotransformation enzymes. These enzymes belong to two phases, aptly named phase I and phase II enzymes. Phase I of liver detox involves the activation of the cytochrome P450 enzymes, which "transform" the toxin and make it more ready for elimination via phase II. After leaving phase I, the new (biotransformed) chemical is shuttled to phase II, where additional work takes place, and the biotransformed chemical is made water soluble—ultimately being kicked out (via bile) into the gastrointestinal tract, or (via kidneys) into urine.

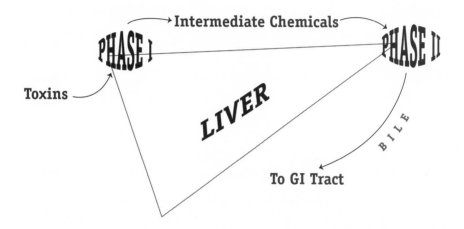

This is the central detox pathway, and when the toxin load is kept to a minimum, stress levels are kept in check, and dietary quality is maximized, all goes well. A proper balance between phase I and phase II is extremely important. Most problems arise when phase II is under-supported. This is particularly bad because when certain relatively benign chemicals are altered (biotransformed) in phase I, the new transformed chemical can actually be more toxic than the original substance! There is also a second problem, which is that the phase I process and the intermediate chemicals generate free radicals. So, with a high toxic load, there is increased activity at phase I and more free radicals being produced and more nasty intermediate chemicals on the loose. If you do not have adequate nutritional support at phase II, you can easily run into trouble. Indeed, many studies show that efficiently operating levels of phase II enzymes are associated with a decreased risk of chemical-induced cancer.

Given that the detox process can cause the generation of free radicals, it is obvious that the intake of dietary antioxidants is of critical importance. In addition, normal functioning of phase I detox is dependent upon nutrients including B vitamins and vitamins C and E. Phase II is highly dependent upon certain amino acids, which are derived from dietary protein. Glutamine and glycine, for example, are critical amino acids in making toxins water soluble for elimination at phase II. In addition, the manufacture of glutathione, arguably the most important antioxidant and phase II detox agent, requires the amino acids glycine, glutamic acid, and cysteine. Higher levels of glutathione have been associated with living a longer and healthier life. Glutathione demand runs high when there is increased toxin load, oxidative stress, inflammation, heavy exercise, and viral infections. Glutathione production slows down in the brain when a chemical called inducible nitric oxide is produced. Given that fish oil, polyphenols, carotenoides, zinc, and taurine can inhibit inducible nitric oxide, all of these dietary factors can indirectly maintain optimal glutathione levels.

With research showing that low levels of glutathione are associated with aging and numerous brain-related conditions from Alzheimer's to schizophrenia, wouldn't it make sense to take glutathione supplements? It would, except that glutathione is not well absorbed by oral administration. When it comes to the manufacture of glutathione via the cellular combining of the three dietary components (glutamine acid, glycine, and cysteine), it is the availability of cysteine which appears to control synthesis. From a dietary perspective, whey protein is very rich in cysteine and has been shown to boost glutathione levels. There is a lot of hype around different types of whey protein, the whole "only ours works" routine. Research published in the *European Journal of Nutrition* (2002) showed that an expensive multilevel-marketed whey protein was actually slightly less effective than another commercially available product at boosting glutathione. When it comes to using cysteine pills as a means to boost glutathione, I would recommend that you save your money. Isolated cysteine may actually promote oxidative stress and act as a toxin to brain cells according to experimental research. N-acetyl-cysteine is a safe alternative to pure cysteine and is used in hospitals to detoxify an acetaminophen overdose. If you take a supplement with N-acetyl-cysteine, keep it to 600 mg or less to avoid adverse effects. Higher doses require supervision by a health-care provider.

Given that many adults have very little trouble with phase I detox and require more support at phase II, taking advantage of foods that specifically induce only phase II enzymes would be an effective way to support optimal detoxification. If you look at the research on the relationship between diet and cancer, vegetables that selectively induce phase II detox enzymes appear to be most protective. One family of plants, the *Brassica* family, emerges as the superstar detox group. The *Brassica* contain chemicals called glucosinolates, which are converted into major phase II detox supporters called isothiocyanates. The bacteria inside your intestinal tract are responsible for this conversion. An important note about the glucosinolates found in *Brassica* veggies is that they are capable of acting in a similar way to drugs that are used for Alzheimer's disease. Drugs used to treat Alzheimer's aim to keep more of the brain neurotransmitter acetylcholine around. Researchers from Kings College London showed that *Brassica* veggies inhibit the enzyme that breaks down acetylcholine, and over the long term it is suggested that they may prevent a decline in levels of acetylcholine within the nervous system.

The *Brassica* Family of Vegetables		
Arugula	Cauliflower	Purple cauliflower
Bok choy	Chinese broccoli	Radish
Broccoli	Daikon	Rutabaga
Broccoli sprouts	Horseradish	Wasabi
Broccolini	Kale	Watercress
Brussels sprouts	Kohlrabi	
Cabbage	Mustard greens	

Drs. Paul Talalay and Jed Fahey of Johns Hopkins University are among the world's leading experts on the influence of the chemicals within *Brassica* plants and detoxification. They have shown that among many grains, meats, dairy, fruits, and non-*Brassica* vegetables, the extracted components didn't even contain 1 percent of the phase II detox activity compared to broccoli. Further, they showed that broccoli, and especially young broccoli sprouts, contain an important chemical called sulforaphane. Canadian researchers showed recently that even a small amount of broccoli sprouts can be protective in the prevention of age-induced nerve degeneration among animals. Writing in the journal *Nutritional Neuroscience* (2005), the researchers from the University of

Saskatoon concluded that even modest changes in diet may have profound effects on the aging within the central nervous system.

Not only does sulforaphane enhance phase II detoxification, it has
been shown to experimentally inhibit the growth of the nasty ulcer-
causing bacteria called *Helicobacter pylori*. In a recent Japanese study published in the journal *Biofactors* (2004), commercially available broccoli
sprouts have been shown to decrease objective markers of oxidative stress
in healthy adults after just one week of consumption. Taking 100 g of
broccoli sprouts lowered total cholesterol, maintained higher levels of the
powerful antioxidant Co-Q10, and decreased 8-isoprostane, a well-
known marker of oxidative stress. Remember that higher 8-isoprostane
levels are associated with a number of brain-related conditions.

As for the anti–*H. pylori* effects of broccoli sprouts, clinical trials are
in the works. An anti–*H. pylori* effect of broccoli sprouts would make
them even more important as part of the Brain Diet plan because
H. pylori bacteria have been associated with both Alzheimer's disease and
migraine headaches. We will explore this in more detail in the next chapter when we discuss the emerging research that shows a relationship
between the bacteria that live in the stomach/intestinal track and brain
health. See the Appendix for information on where you can get broccoli
sprouts.

In addition to the *Brassica* vegetables, there are other dietary components that can support phase II detoxification. Onions, garlic, green tea,
pomegranates, Thai ginger, honey, and leeks can also help with normal
detoxification. Turmeric (curcumin) is also a rising star, as are some of the
components of citrus. The bottom line is that the ultimate detox diet is
not all that different from that which has been promoted for cardiovascular disease and general health—one with a variety of fruits and vegetables. Based on the emerging science, detox can be maximized by
including *Brassica* vegetables, and broccoli sprouts in particular. Cooking
with turmeric, ginger, and other spices, as well as drinking green tea, can
add to the cumulative effect.

As mentioned, fiber is also an important concept in detox. Since the
majority of environmental toxins enter the body via food and water, it
would make sense to reduce absorption at the intestinal level. We discussed already that the integrity of the intestinal lining is essential in
this regard. Dietary fiber, including rice bran and wheat bran, has been

shown to help bind up and remove environmental toxins. In one study rice bran enhanced the excretion of dioxins and PCBs at two to three times the rate of the nonfibrous control. Wheat bran has been shown to effectively bind to mercury, cadmium, and lead and therefore diminish absorption and negative consequence. Given that weight loss increases circulating toxins, it should follow that any long-term weight-loss program should be one high in fiber. In addition to the binding of chemicals, fiber also promotes the growth of beneficial bacteria that in turn enhance detox.

In animal studies, fish oil has been shown to accelerate the excretion of environmental organochlorine chemicals. As we already discussed, fish oil enhances weight loss in animals, and when that happens the environmental chemicals that are stored in fat cells are set free. However, the mobilized toxins may actually prevent the breakdown and use of fat as an energy source. Taking fish oil turns on phase I enzymes, which help metabolize chemicals and get rid of them. Support at phase II from other dietary factors would likely enhance the detox role of fish oil. Hopefully human studies will further investigate the role of different fats on weight control and environmental toxins.

With regard to environmental molds, there is one dietary agent that may limit the associated symptoms. Writing in the *Archives of Environmental Health* (2003), Dr. Sherry Rogers has outlined a number of mechanisms whereby alpha-lipoic acid may be helpful in dealing with the symptoms of mold exposure. Alpha-lipoic acid is a commercially available supplement and is known as the universal antioxidant, as it is both water and fat soluble and protects against all kinds of free radicals. Alpha-lipoic acid may be particularly effective in preventing free radical damage in the brain.

When it comes to detoxification in the liver, any kind of prolonged fasting beyond one day is completely inappropriate. The detoxification system relies upon proteins and other dietary chemicals for optimal function. While intermittent fasting may have its place in human health and brain function, we need much more research before it can be routinely recommended. The Environmental Working Group (www.ewg.org) is the place to go for the most updated and unbiased source of information regarding pesticides and contaminants in our foods. They have no agenda other than to support human health and wellness. Here, from the EWG,

Most Contaminated Foods	Least Contaminated Foods
Apples	Asparagus
Bell peppers	Avocado
Celery	Banana
Cherries	Broccoli
Grapes (imported)	Cauliflower
Nectarines	Corn
Peaches	Kiwi
Pears	Mango
Potatoes	Onions
Red raspberries	Papaya
Spinach	Pineapple
Strawberries	Peas

are the most pesticide-contaminated fruits and vegetables, as well as those that pose little risk.

Organic foods can be expensive, and while making efforts to choose only organic foods is worthwhile for our greater good, it is not always practical. The Brain Diet plan suggests that the fruits and vegetables with the highest amounts of pesticides should be avoided and replaced with organic choices. In considering which fruits and vegetables to prioritize, be guided by the lists above and any updated information provided by the Environmental Working Group.

There have been some small studies on the combination of commercially available detoxification supplements and elimination diets (removal of potentially sensitive foods such as wheat and dairy). The products generally include dietary nutrients such as green tea, N-acetyl-cysteine, and other antioxidant and anti-inflammatory food-based ingredients. These studies have shown that such combinations enhance liver detox and reduce the symptoms of those with chronic fatigue syndrome and fibromyalgia.

Detoxification food supplements that also require the removal of specific allergenic foods should be used under the supervision of a health-care professional. It certainly makes enormous sense to remove foods high in chemicals and make efforts to choose organic foods to lower the toxin load. However, when it comes to the investigation of foods that potentially cause food intolerances and contribute to fatigue, mood alterations, and cognitive disturbances, this requires guidance because there is potential for nutritional deficiencies to occur.

Food intolerances are separate and distinct from the classic (called IgE) food allergy—the potentially life-threatening kind, with severe allergies to peanuts, shellfish, strawberries, etc. Food intolerances are vague in symptom presentation, less intense, and may come on sometime after the food or beverage has been consumed. Typical symptoms of food intolerance might be headaches, brain fog or cognitive difficulties, anxiety, hyperactivity, and fatigue.

As you might imagine with these types of symptoms and no recognized laboratory test, those with food intolerances are often dismissed as having only psychiatric problems. In desperation, they often end up in the offices of alternative medicine practitioners who use all kinds of fancy machines to "uncover" food intolerances. I bring this up now because many Web sites, books, and articles recommend limiting food or trying to evaluate food sensitivities (via pseudoscientific gadgets) as part of detox protocols.

The machines purported to uncover food intolerances have various trade names, but most are one form or another of so-called "electro-

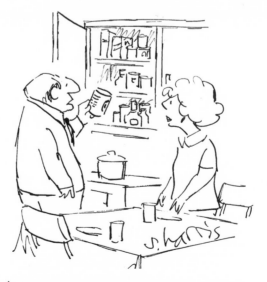

" 'CLAM CHOWDER—INGREDIENTS: CLAMS, POTATOES,
WATER, HYDROLATED PLANT PROTEIN, SODIUM
PHOSPHATE, CALCIUM CARBONATE, BUTYLATED
HYDROXYTOLUNE. FOR EXTERNAL USE ONLY.' "

dermal screening." Operators claim they can determine allergies and sensitivities by running a pen-like device over the end of your finger. Patients get a fancy paper printout of (usually many) foods to avoid— and they may, or may not, receive dietary counseling on appropriate food substitutes.

It would be great if electro-dermal screening worked, but despite the testimonials and commercial literature, research shows that it is of no value at all. Two well-designed studies, one in the *British Medical Journal* (2001), and the other in *Clinical and Experimental Allergy* (2002), found that these devices were unable to "uncover" allergies. It is not that they just lighten up the wallet, there is a real danger in these machines, given the sheer number of foods that consumers are advised to eliminate. I had one chronic fatigue patient who showed me a list of more than fifty foods that she was told to avoid, simply because the machine and printout said so. The patient was basically cajoled into an eating disorder. In patients who are already anxious, there is then a great fear instilled regarding the reintroduction of foods into the diet, and obviously nutritional deficiencies can occur when you eliminate long lists of foods. When you list as many as fifty possibilities, it is highly likely that you have indeed "uncovered" the one or two foods (usually wheat, dairy, or citrus) that were causing the problem; this, in turn, makes the operator and the patient feel somewhat better and reinforces the notion (for both) that the machine is a genius.

I do need to point out that food intolerance is a real entity, and if you have a list of vague symptoms that have been properly evaluated with no medical explanation, then a supervised elimination diet may be helpful. The vague brain-related symptoms of food intolerance were given a real credibility boost thanks to a landmark study in the prestigious journal *Lancet* (2000). Dr. Morten Jacobsen and colleagues from the University of Oslo, Norway, showed that those with food intolerances (not classic food allergy) have a significant elevation in inflammatory cytokines when they are challenged with intolerant foods, in this case wheat and dairy. As the researchers pointed out, it was a connection that could explain the many symptoms of food sensitivity.

Remember the cytokines? They are the immune chemicals that, when elevated in otherwise healthy adults, can cause anxiety, depression, and cognitive difficulties. This incredible research challenges

• • • CASE REPORT • • •

Anne is a thirty-four-year-old lawyer who complained of fatigue, poor sleep, and a variety of gastrointestinal disturbances. She had noticed these symptoms progress over the previous two years. Anne formerly relished her work as an attorney; however, the fatigue and lack of mental focus were compromising her ability to perform to her usual standards. This in turn made her view work as a pressure-filled and stressful environment.

The first steps were to get Anne's diet corrected. Like many North Americans, she had been running on low-grade dietary fuel including fast foods and soft drinks. Fried foods and sandwiches with processed meat were also a large part of her dietary picture, while fish was nonexistent. More recently, Anne had turned to canned energy drinks for a morning and afternoon boost.

Deeply colored fruits and vegetables were incorporated into her diet and whole grains were emphasized as a staple for energy. A daily multivitamin and an omega-3 fatty acid supplement were also recommended, as she was not fond of fish. Breakfast with at least one whole-grain item became routine, and this provided Anne with a sustainable lift in energy through the morning. The afternoon energy drink, containing almost 30 g of sugar per can, was replaced with greens+™, a plant-food based nutritional product shown in University of Toronto research to boost energy in otherwise healthy adults.

In addition to dietary modifications and the two supplements, the use of mind-body interventions and the relaxation response in particular were effective in keeping Anne away from negative "future-thinking." As Anne's energy and mental focus improved, she became less stressed at work and her sleep quality improved without the use of medications.

the notion that food intolerances are solely psychological. If you feel that food intolerances might be affecting your mood or mental edge, pass on the unscientific machines and non-validated blood tests and work with your health-care provider the old fashioned way—elimination and reintroduction (challenge) one at a time. Research shows that use of a food and symptom diary can help to identify problem foods.

Summary

Exposure to environmental toxins has become part of our modern existence. Whether one lives in an urban or rural environment, excessive accumulation of toxins in human tissue is a reality. Emerging research is showing that environmental toxins have the potential to influence genetic expression, and to influence neurological and psychiatric symptoms.

Pesticides, heavy metals, food colors, preservatives, and aerosolized molds are just a few of the chemicals that may influence brain chemistry, physiology, and ultimately behavior. To make matters worse, there may be a synergistic activity of environmental toxins when they act together. In addition, stress, infections, and background health can influence the extent to which environmental toxins exert their effects. Toxins stored in the body and released upon weight loss may actually slow metabolism, prevent the further breakdown of fat, and encourage weight gain.

Waste management is an extremely important concept in brain health. We must provide adequate nutritional support to our liver and gastrointestinal tract. The old traditional detox, with harsh botanical remedies and such, is an outdated and questionable concept in today's world. We need continuous nutritional support of our detoxification systems. Certain dietary items can provide that nutritional support. *Brassica* vegetables, probiotics, green tea, rice bran and other fiber, antioxidants, alpha-lipoic acid, and taurine are among some of the important players in the detoxification system. High-quality whey protein and N-acetyl-cysteine can also provide a boost in glutathione, arguably our most important liver detoxifying and antioxidant chemical.

Food intolerances may play an underappreciated role in the various cognitive and mood-related symptoms in those with certain brain disorders. The intolerances may be to the actual food, or to the chemicals added to it. Either way, an investigation using a supervised elimination and re-challenge diet may be worthwhile.

Now let's have a look at the exciting research connecting the health of the gut with the health of our brain.

6

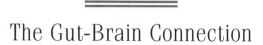

The Gut-Brain Connection

FROM THE MOMENT YOU TAKE your first breath of air and begin life on this planet, the once-sterile environment of your gastrointestinal tract (GI) is being colonized by bacteria. As life goes on, more and more bacteria will set up camp in your intestines until you have about 100,000,000,000,000 bacteria belonging to more than four hundred different species. The overwhelming majority of these bacteria reside not in the stomach and small intestine, but inside the large intestine, also known as the colon. Normal intestinal bacteria are referred to as microflora, and every minute of every day, without your even being aware, they are defending your health. The microflora have a profound effect on your immune system and, as we discussed in the last chapter, they play an important role in the intestinal barrier, keeping the riff-raff of toxins and bad bacteria on the outside.

While the influence of the intestinal microflora on general health has been known for many years, it is only recently that researchers have been making some connections with the brain. Most of the research over the years was limited to the local effects of intestinal bacteria on digestive disorders. As we will discuss, there is now ample evidence to suggest that the living inhabitants of your GI tract can play an important role in longevity, brain health, mood, and behavior. Among the many bacterial species that reside in the GI tract, two are of real importance to human health. *Lactobacilli* and *Bifidobacteria*, the so-called friendly bacteria, are involved in vitamin synthesis, the detoxification and metabolism of toxic substances, stimulation of the immune response, protection from patho-genic (bad) bacteria, and the defense of the intestinal lining. In addition, *Lactobacilli* and *Bifidobacteria* can lower levels of brain-toxic compounds that can otherwise build up through digestive and other metabolic processes. While many mainstream gastroenterologists and neurologists would be quick to dismiss the functioning of *Lactobacilli* and *Bifidobacteria* as being of no relevance to brain function and behavior, emerging research supports a connection. Recently, bacteria belonging to these genera have been shown to lower immune cytokine levels, not only locally in the gut, but also in the body-wide bloodstream when orally administered. This systemic effect is so pronounced that the beneficial bacteria (so-called probiotics) are capable of reducing joint inflammation in arthritic rats. As we have discussed, these cytokines, including TNF alpha and IL-6, are the very same chemicals that when induced in healthy adults cause anxiety, depressive symptoms, and cognitive distur-bances. These same cytokines can lower levels of brain-derived neu-rotrophic factor (BDNF), our old friend and protector of our nerve cells.

The body-wide effect of oral probiotics on inflammatory cytokines is impressive, but it is by no means the only way in which probiotics can influence brain and behavior. In fact, I'm just getting started. Recent studies also show that species from these genera act as major antioxidants. At least four impressive studies have shown that probiotics are protective against free radical damage, particularly against damage to the lipid (fat) component of cells. In one incredible study by Dr. Tatyana Oxman and colleagues from Israel, orally administered *Lactobacillus bulgaricus* was shown to protect heart cells against the effects of ischemia (lack of oxy-genated blood supply). The protective effects were most likely related to an antioxidant effect. The studies are not limited only to test tubes and animals; in one impressive study, published in the *American Journal of Clinical Nutrition* (2003), Swedish researchers showed that a strain of *Lactobacillus plantarum*, identified as 299v, could improve cardiovascular risk factors in smokers. Specifically, they showed that oral administration of the bacteria lowered blood pressure and blood markers associated with cardiovascular disease. Of real importance regarding brain health, the researchers showed a 37 percent reduction in the F-isoprostanes. If you recall, they are the markers of oxidative stress, the chemicals that are ele-vated in many neurodenerative diseases. In addition, the *Lactobacillus plantarum* 299V group had a 42 percent reduction in blood levels of the inflammatory cytokine called IL-6. This is an important immune chemi-cal that has the potential to influence mood and cognition in a negative way. There is no question that the bacteria residing in the intestinal tract can have far-reaching effects, way beyond the gut. Amazing—tiny microbes capable of lowering oxidative stress and inflammatory chemi-cals outside of the gut. As you will see, when it comes to the Brain Diet, a few select probiotics should be part of the plan.

Consider also a 2003 study in the *American Journal of Clinical Nutrition* where it was demonstrated that oral consumption of commer-cially available *Lactobacillus* GG was shown to lower the levels of unde-sirable bacteria in the nasal cavity. Specifically, the group consuming *Lactobacillus* GG had a significant reduction in the type of bacteria that will ordinarily send you and your children to the doctor for sinusitis or otitis (ear infection). This doctor visit often results in a prescription for an antibiotic. I bring this up because the overprescription of antibiotics is appalling. At one time antibiotics were prescribed like candy, and although things have improved, they are still grossly over-used. Antibiotics are now being associated with the onset of a number of human conditions, including irritable bowel syndrome, Crohn's disease, breast cancer, allergies, and asthma. The common thread among all of these conditions is alterations in intestinal microflora. Up to 85 percent of antibiotic prescriptions for sore throats, coughs, and colds are uncalled for. The long-term impact of antibiotics on intestinal microflora is well known, but only recently has the importance of maintaining a healthy gut flora been given scientific support. Antibiotics should be reserved for the times when they are really needed, and if the overprescription is not curtailed, they will be much less likely to work when we need them to. The issue of antibiotic resistance by smart bacteria is becoming a global concern. Not only can antibiotics kill off beneficial bacteria, which do so much for us, the bacteria are replaced by other undesirable organisms, like yeast, which are unaffected by antibiotics.

Yeasts, including *Candida albicans*, can produce alcohol and stimulate the release of inflammatory chemicals. In addition, yeasts contain many antigens that resemble food-based protein; this can lead to the initiation of food intolerances in those with yeast overgrowth in the GI tract. In a placebo-controlled study published in the journal *Family Practice* (2001), antifungal therapy improved the symptoms of those with unexplained medical illness—the usual constellation of symptoms that normally gets one referred to a psychiatrist. Specifically, the antifungal medication (Nystatin) taken orally (versus placebo) improved brain-related symptoms including mood swings, anxiety, brain fog, feelings of unreality, fatigue, drained feeling, memory dysfunction, insomnia, depression, and inability to make decisions.

There is also some exciting new research which has uncovered a beautiful relationship between beneficial bacteria and omega-3 fatty acids. Research shows that all types of dietary fats do not have the same effect when it comes to influencing the growth of intestinal bacteria. Japanese researchers showed that among three different diets (one high in omega-6 corn oil, another high in beef fat, and a third high in fish oil), it was the fish oil group that showed a beneficial effect on intestinal flora. Specifically, the fish oil diet led to a threefold increase in *Bifidobacteria* and the lowest levels of the *Bacteroides* group of bacteria. This is significant because *Bacteroides* are implicated in cancer. Separate experimental research has shown that a diet high in fish oil or flaxseed oil, both rich in omega-3, can increase *Lactobacilli*. In contrast, coconut oil, high in saturated fats, does not increase beneficial bacteria. In addition, test-tube studies have shown that omega-6–rich corn oil and pure linoleic acid itself (parent omega-6 oil) are both inhibitory to the growth of *Bifidobacteria*. Pure EPA from fish oil, on the other hand, is inhibitory to human *Bacteroides*.

Beyond the increase in the growth of beneficial bacteria, the polyunsaturated fats appear to influence the adhesion of good bacteria to the intestinal wall. Arachidonic acid is found in beef fat, and it is also produced from the omega-6 vegetable oils we are overconsuming. Arachidonic acid causes less adhesion of good bacteria to intestinal cells, while flaxseed oil, rich in omega-3, increases the adhesion of bacteria. Marine oils, high in EPA, have been shown to markedly increase the adhesion of *Lactobacillus* to the intestines.

Published reports as far back as 1964 have shown that olive oil can increase numbers of *Lactobacillus*. Researchers are just now beginning to understand how different lipids might influence the adhesion of bacteria.

Incredibly, fatty acids are actually taken up inside the bacteria and have the potential to alter bacterial structures, and therefore the adhesion to our intestines as well. Now, as I mentioned, this is a beautiful relationship, and not one where it is take, take, take on the part of selfish *Lactobacillus* and *Bifidobacteria*—research shows that the relationship is a two-way street with give and take. When researchers from Finland examined the role of oral *Bifidobacteria* administration to allergic children, not only did they find benefit, they also noted an increase in the parent omega-3 fatty acid, alpha-linolenic acid. Further hints come from a McGill University study where hens that had a *Lactobacillus* probiotic blend mixed into their flaxseed-containing food had higher levels of EPA in eggs versus flaxseed-based food alone. It really makes you think about the synergy of food and bacteria.

Consider Japan. The oldest living people on the planet reside there, and it is a place where depression, seasonal affective disorders, violent acts, and neurodegenerative diseases occur much less frequently. Researchers from the University of Tokyo and the Ludwig Institute of Cancer in Toronto compared the fecal microflora of Japanese residents consuming a typical Japanese diet to that of healthy Torontonians consuming a typical Western diet. As you may have already guessed, the levels of *Lactobacilli* and *Bifidobacteria* were significantly higher among the Japanese. In contrast the Canadians had much higher levels of the *Bacteroides* (cancer suspects) and various *Clostridium* species (autism suspects).

The Japanese diet contains elements that are known to positively influence intestinal microflora. Take, for example, green tea. Research shows that green tea promotes the growth of *Bifidobacteria*, and incredibly, the EGCG component has been shown to enhance the effectiveness of antifungal medications against *Candida*. In fact, the most pronounced effect of EGCG from green tea was against drug resistant *Candida* strains. It has also been reported that ginger has strong antimicrobial properties, but may contribute to the growth of *Lactobacilli*. Honey is also a great way to sweeten foods because it contains antioxidant polyphenols, and at least two studies have shown that it can selectively promote the growth of *Bifidobacteria* and *Lactobacilli*. The dietary fiber, the omega-3 fatty acids from fish, the green tea, and a host of other colorful phytonutrients within the Japanese diet may influence intestinal microflora in a beneficial way.

Even within Japan, adherence to a higher-fiber traditional diet can influence the intestinal bacteria. In an eye-opening study published in *Applied and Environmental Microbiology* (1989), researchers from the University of Tokyo showed that those living in the rural Yuzurihara/Yamanashi regions had a different intestinal microflora profile from those living in urban Tokyo. What was so special about this is that the Yazurihara/Yamanashi regions are known as the residence of some of the longest-lived individuals in Japan. Given that the Japanese are the longest-living people on the planet, a close look at the Yuzurihara/Yamanashi region would of course be worthwhile. The overall levels of *Bifidobacteria* were much higher in the rural, long-lived region versus Tokyo. In addition, there were much lower levels of the problematic *Clostridium* and *Bacteroides* groups.

The levels of *Bifidobacteria* are well known to drop down with advancing age. The levels of *Bifidobacteria* in the rural region, where residents adhere more strictly to the traditional Japanese diet, were higher than that of a Tokyo resident twenty years younger. In particular, one species of *Bifidobacteria* is actually emerging as a marker for aging. *Bifidobacteria adolescentis* levels drop off in a linear fashion with the aging process. The researchers found that this particular bacteria, *B. adolescentis*, was much higher in elderly persons living in the Yuzurihara/Yamanashi region. Of course this does not translate into *B. adolescentis* being a fountain of youth bacteria. However, the loss of *Bifidobacteria* means a gain in the *Clostridium* and *Bacteroides* groups, which in turn can elevate the manufacture of brain-toxic protein breakdown products.

Remember when we talked about the detoxifying potential of broccoli sprouts, wasabi, and other *Brassica* family vegetables? Well, it turns out that these guys have selective effects on intestinal microbial inhabitants. Broccoli sprouts and wasabi in particular are known inhibitors of the nasty stomach bacteria *Helicobacter pylori*, the one involved in the formation of ulcers. Yet wasabi and broccoli sprouts appear to leave *Lactobacilli* and *Bifidobacteria* alone. This diet and *H. pylori* connection has some real brain ramifications. Consider that *H. pylori* infection has been associated with a greater risk of Alzheimer's disease, higher frequency of migraine headaches, and higher levels of pain at distant sites in irritable bowel syndrome.

It is quite incredible that bacteria in the stomach can influence pain at sites far removed from where the bacteria actually reside. It is downright unbelievable that *H. pylori* infection could be related to later Alzheimer's disease, but that is what research published in the *European Journal of Internal Medicine* (2004) suggests. The chronic, low-level inflammation that is initiated and maintained by *H. pylori* may be the culprit. A growing number of experimental studies have shown that various strains of probiotic bacteria can inhibit the growth of *H. pylori*. The suppressive effect of probiotics on *H. pylori* may result from the production of direct antimicrobial chemicals secreted by the good bacteria, and it may also be related to the *Lactobacilli* provoking an enhanced immune response. In addition to the test-tube and animal studies, at least four human studies have shown that various strains of *Lactobacillus* have a pronounced anti–*H. pylori* effect. Two additional studies show that probiotics can cut down on the side effects such as diarrhea, nausea, and taste disturbance in those taking conventional antibiotics for *H. pylori*. With this backdrop, researchers from the L Sacco Teaching Hospital in Milan, Italy, investigated the effects of probiotics on migraine patients with *H. pylori*. It was a large enough study, with more than 130 participants who were split into an antibiotic group and an antibiotic plus *Lactobacillus* group. Despite similar headache frequency and bacterial numbers at baseline, some interesting findings were noted at the one-year follow-up. When re-evaluated, 40 percent of the antibiotic group were *H. pylori*–free, compared to 70 percent in the antibiotic plus probiotic group. Here is where it gets really good—both the severity and frequency of migraine headaches were reduced among those in the probiotic group. The study leaves us with more questions than answers, but certainly adds kerosene to the gut-brain connection fire.

Autointoxication

The term *intestinal autointoxication* refers to the notion that some diseases can arise from toxins produced within the gastrointestinal tract. It is hardly a modern concept; even the ancient Egyptians suggested that a toxic agent associated with the feces was related to disease. In the 1800s, with the advancement of science, some theorized that the decomposition of proteins in the intestines (termed putrefaction) could cause illness and disease. In 1880, Lauder Brunton of the United Kingdom suggested that imperfect digestion and protein fermentation could cause nervous depression. Hydrogen sulfide produced by protein breakdown was held responsible for intestinal harm. Other investigators throughout Europe were making similar suggestions. Constipation became vilified and the root of all illness. With the advances of modern surgery, in 1893, Dr. William Lane started to advocate "bypassing" and cutting out the colon by surgical means. The rationale was of course to prevent constipation, which he attributed to everything from skin wrinkling to depression, from irritability to dementia. Ultimately Lane considered constipation to be related to premature aging.

Ellie Metchnikoff, winner of the Nobel Prize of Medicine in 1908, also suggested that premature aging was related to toxins from the gut, but his solution was not to cut out the colon—he advocated altering the intestinal microflora. He theorized that intestinal putrefaction produced toxins that shortened life span. Basically, food residues are broken down, or putrefied, by intestinal bacteria in the colon. Among Europeans at that time, the Bulgarians, the Turks, and the Armenians had notable longevity. When he looked closely at the diets of all three groups, the frequent consumption of fermented milk was the common thread. Specifically, two bacteria were identified in fermented milk, *Lactobacillus bulgaricus*, and *Streptococcus thermophilus*. These bacteria could inhibit the bacteria involved in putrefaction.

In the early 1900s, scientists identified the chemicals produced from protein putrefaction in the intestines. Chemicals such as indoles and skatoles became major culprits, as both can increase with protein fermentation. However, by the end of the 1920s some researchers called the idea of autointoxication nonsense, and some studies showed that constipation and putrefactive chemicals had no bearing on human illness. The theory went down like a lead balloon. When researchers showed that experimental distention of the rectum could cause the symptoms associated with constipation, such as abdominal pain and discomfort, the autointoxication movement drifted away.

In modern medical journals, autointoxication is mentioned mostly in the context of historical articles. Most modern historical examinations are often smug and arrogant, and almost never consider that autointoxication theories have resulted in modern disease connections. Today, autointoxication is brought up in medical journals mainly to look back and have a laugh about how "wrong" everybody was at the turn of the last century. But were they really wrong about everything? Did they not contribute to our understanding of some incredible connections between what happens inside the gut and what may happen in areas far removed from it?

The old autointoxication theories were undoubtedly associated with drastic measures such as surgery and drinking paraffin oil to get the bowels moving, or antiseptics to purify the colon. Still, thanks to further advances in science we now know that high consumption of red meat is associated with colon cancer and ulcerative colitis. We know that red meat undergoes putrefaction by bacteria such as *E. coli*, *Clostridium*, and *Bacteroides* groups. Writing in the *Journal of Gastroenterology and Hepatology* (2003), researchers from the Shiga University of Medical Sciences in Japan showed that indole and other potentially toxic putrefactive substances such as spermidine, putrescine, and spermine are indeed well absorbed from the intestinal tract and into circulation.

While low levels of protein breakdown products (polyamines) from putrefaction are actually beneficial in the growth of intestinal cells, and in the brain for memory consolidation, elevated levels of polyamines are now also known to be toxic to brain cells and are associated with colon cancer. High blood levels of one putrefaction product, spermidine, have been observed in patients with schizophrenia and excess intestinal absorption is thought to play a role.

Consider also that inadequate dietary folate leads to elevations in blood levels of putrefactive polyamines. Researchers from the University of Saskatchewan, Canada, showed that mild folate deficiency elevated blood polyamine levels by 27 percent. Remember that folate has been shown to be critical to mood and memory, with low levels now clearly connected to depression and cognitive decline. Stress can also increase blood and brain levels of polyamines, an increase that can be prevented by the administration of anti-anxiety medications. Although the brain can manufacture some of its own polyamines, the influence of dietary factors in this process certainly deserves attention.

Putrefactive substances such as indole accumulate in the intestines when aerobic bacteria rapidly multiply (overgrowth) and set up camp. An overgrowth of aerobic bacteria in the GI tract is thought to be responsible for the development of food intolerances. Active chemicals produced by the overgrown bacteria acting upon food may lead to cytokine elevations.

We also now know that hydrogen sulfide (H_2S) production is increased inside the colon with elevated consumption of meats, and we know now that hydrogen sulfide is a major player in the development of ulcerative colitis. H_2S gas production is also a feature of bacterial overgrowth in the intestines. H_2S gas can then enter the blood. Although hydrogen sulfide gas is normally readily excreted by the lungs, an effect on the brain over time may be a factor in brain-related symptoms in those with chronic intestinal disorders. H_2S entering the lungs, even at tiny amounts (125 parts in one million), has been shown to reduce learning and memory in adult animals. When it comes to learning and memory, H_2S increases the susceptibility to interference from irrelevant environmental stimuli. Animals and modern, overstimulated humans have difficulty sorting out what information should be prioritized and what information should be dismissed. In human research, exposure to H_2S has been associated with both cognitive and emotional disturbances.

The autointoxication movement was far from wrong, far from a folly. It was certainly taken to extremes, but many of the original theories are now being validated, particularly those related to intestinal bacteria and fiber. Ultimately, constipation may be a marker for low intake of dietary fiber. This, in turn, may be suggestive of a diet low in nutrient-dense foods. While there may be confounding factors, some studies have shown that constipation is associated with a greater risk of colon and breast cancer.

As the research advances, we are beginning to see that the real joke is on those who arrogantly dismissed autointoxication so easily just a decade ago. Thanks to new research published in the journal *Digestive and Liver Disease* (2005), we now know that chronic constipation is associated with significant changes in the intestinal microflora (lower beneficial *Lactobacillus* and *Bifidobacteria*) and a sharp increase in intestinal permeability. It is also associated with an elevation in body-wide immune system activity—i.e., chronic constipation provokes an unnecessary immune response way beyond the local GI tract, likely because unwanted materials gain body-wide access through a more permeable intestinal tract. Given that low-grade inflammation is characteristic of this body-wide immune response, and that chronic low-grade inflammation is a major player in cardiovascular disease and most brain-related conditions, the importance of this new research cannot be overstated.

Some interesting research shows that constipation predates any observable movement-related symptoms of Parkinson's disease by up to twenty years. It has been hypothesized that toxins that gain access through the intestinal barrier enter directly into the nervous system. Japanese researchers, writing in the *Journal of Neurology* (2004), showed that the decreased intake of water was directly associated with pre-illness constipation, and that decreased water intake was noted from early life, decades before Parkinson's set in. On the other hand, coffee, a beverage known to stimulate bowel movements, has been shown to be protective against Parkinson's disease.

Modern research has also allowed us to see that specific bacteria within the intestinal tract can influence the motility (or propulsion) of food and waste matter. Researchers have shown that *Lactobacilli* and *Bifidobacteria* actually speed things up and promote the transit of material through the intestines. *E. coli,* on the other hand, a bacteria that can ferment proteins and produce toxic chemicals, actually slows down movement. It would then seem plausible that the oral delivery of probiotic strains might improve constipation. In a landmark study in the *Canadian Journal of Gastroenterology* (2003), researchers showed that *Lactobacillus casei* strain Shirota has a highly significant effect in improving chronic constipation. Compared to placebo, the *Lactobacillus casei* Shirota (consumed as a beverage called Yakult) group showed significant improvement in both stool consistency and bowel movements. Positive effects were noted about two weeks into the one-month study. In the final analysis, 89 percent of those in the Yakult group experienced improvement in constipation versus about half in the placebo group. Such effects may be specific to this particular strain of bacteria, so I am pleased to say that the Yakult drink has finally made its way to the shores of North America (see the Appendix for details). *Lactobacillus casei* strain Shirota has been consumed in the form of Yakult beverages for the better part of the last century. Yakult is widely acclaimed and is perhaps the most recognizable commercial drink in Japan; from young children to the elderly, almost everyone has had a Yakult. If you need one more reason to take Yakult on a regular basis, consider a 2005 study in the *Journal of the Neurological Sciences* in which Japanese researchers showed that taking *Lactobacillus*

casei strain Shirota for one month improved the symptoms of a viral-
induced neurological condition characterized by progressive weakness,
sensory disturbances, and urinary dysfunction. This study underscores,
once again, the undervalued connection between the gut bacteria and
the goings-on in the nervous system.

Just one more note on protein fermentation and autointoxication
before we move on: certain types of bacteria that act upon dietary proteins produce chemicals that can add to the body burden of oxidative
stress. For example, the amino acid (protein) tyrosine is acted upon by
Clostridium species to form p-cresol, a chemical that depletes our most
important antioxidant and liver detox chemical called glutathione. The
p-cresol formed by the action of *Clostridium* also induces free radical damage in lipid (fat) structures. The amino acid tryptophan can be targeted
by *E. coli*'s bacterial enzymes to produce indole, which, as mentioned, is
absorbed through the intestines and converted into toxic indolxyl sulfate.
High levels of indolxyl sulfate, otherwise known as indican, have been
associated with neurological and psychiatric symptoms. In contrast,
Bifidobacteria do not have tryptophanase (enzyme that acts on tryptophan) activity and are not involved in the production of p-cresol and
indican. Researchers from Nagoya University Hospital in Japan have
published a number of studies showing that orally administered
Bifidobacteria can actually lower levels of indican. Higher levels of
Lactobacillus strains are also associated with lower urinary indican.

Dr. Henry Butt and colleagues from the University of Newcastle,
Australia, showed that higher aerobic (air-loving) bacteria in the gut are
associated with a host of gastrointestinal symptoms. One aerobic bacterial group, *Enterococcus* species, were much higher in the more than 1,300
subjects with persistent, medically unexplained fatigue. The patients,
most of whom met the criteria for chronic fatigue syndrome, irritable
bowl syndrome, and fibromyalgia, had low levels of *Bifidobacteria*.
Amazingly, the higher the individual (aerobic) *Enterococci* levels, the
more severe were the neurological and cognitive dysfunctions. For example, those with high levels of *Enterococci* were more likely to be nervous,
forgetful, confused, and complaining of memory loss. More fuel for the
gut-brain fire?

Small Intestinal Bacteria Overgrowth

Irritable bowel syndrome, endometriosis, chronic fatigue syndrome, and fibromyalgia (IBS, EM, CFS, FM) have at least three common threads—low levels of beneficial bacteria, depressive symptoms, and the overgrowth of bacteria in the small intestine. Note that the small intestine is home to relatively few bacteria when someone is in good health. When stomach acid becomes low due to aging and/or continuous antacid medications, this allows bacteria to migrate upward from the colon and set up camp in the small intestine. This overgrowth can also occur when there is a lack of motility in the GI tract, when things remain stagnant as in constipation. Physical inactivity, common to depression, aging, and the aforementioned conditions, can also compromise motility and set the stage for bacterial overgrowth in the small intestine. While small intestinal bacterial overgrowth (SIBO) has not been formally investigated in depression, it is highly likely to occur. Patients with depression are known to have low levels of stomach acid production and intestinal stasis (stagnation due to poor motility). In fact, the very cytokines implicated in depression, IL-1 beta and TNF alpha, are capable of inhibiting stomach acid secretion.

Symptoms of SIBO can include bloating, abdominal pain, constipation, diarrhea, gas, and even fatigue and pain distant from the intestinal sites. University of Toronto physician and researcher Dr. Martin Katzman, and myself, have proposed that the symptoms of SIBO may also enter the mental realm. With bacteria encroaching into an area where the majority of digestion occurs, it should not be surprising that SIBO patients have difficulty with proper absorption of proteins, fats, carbohydrates, B vitamins, and other nutrients due to bacterial interference. Bacteria in the small intestine can successfully compete for nutrients known to regulate mood, and they can produce toxic products, and cause direct injury to the intestinal cells.

Dr. Mark Pimentel of Cedars-Sinai Medical Center in Los Angeles is one of the world's leading authorities on SIBO. It was his team that first made solid scientific connections between IBS and bacterial overgrowth in the small intestine. Dr. Pimentel's group has had short-term success treating SIBO with antibiotics. In one particular study, the treatment of SIBO in CFS patients with antibiotics was shown to influence brain and nervous-system symptoms. The study, published in the journal *Gastroenterology* (2000), showed that medical reduction of bacterial over-growth in the small intestine improved symptoms of depression, memory and concentration.

Interestingly, various stains of *Lactobacillus* and *Bifidobacteria* have been documented to be of value in the treatment of SIBO. This positive effect is most likely to be due to the fact that such bacteria can get the bowels moving and prevent the stasis which can be at the root of the prob-lem. In addition, my col-league Dr. Tracey Beaulne of the Integrative Care Centre of Toronto has had clinical success treating SIBO with enteric-coated capsules of essential oils. Peppermint, oregano, anise, garlic, and thyme oils, as well as cran-berry, have been shown to

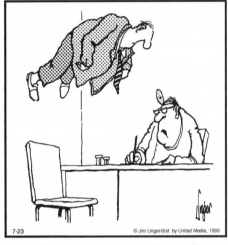

HERMAN®

7-23   © Jim Unger/dist. by United Media, 1999

"I'll give you something for gas."

have antibacterial and anti-*Candida* properties in experimental studies. In addition, some clinicians recommend encapsulated hydrochloric acid (HCl) to help with digestion and prevent microbes from setting up camp in the small intestine. Peppermint oil has been shown in a number of studies to be of value in IBS, and it does appear to have a regulating effect on intestinal motility.

I am reluctant to recommend potent antibiotics for SIBO, only because they have been associated with the onset of IBS and other condi-tions. A new non-absorbable antibiotic, Rifaximin, which acts only in the GI tract, has been reported to be more appropriate and clinically useful in eradication of SIBO. More recently, Dr. Pimentel and colleagues have been using an elemental dietary formulation (Vivonex Plus, Novartis Nutrition), a nutritionally complete liquid meal that is absorbed within the first portion of the small intestine. This starves the majority of bacte-ria in the small intestines and they die off. It is known that fasting can do the same thing, but this liquid meal is obviously a better way to go.

Elemental diets have been shown to be helpful in Crohn's disease as well, with documented reductions in gastrointestinal inflammation. Research also shows that the elemental diets can significantly reduce *E. coli*, *Enterococci*, *Clostridium*, and *Bacteroides* groups—yes, the very bacteria that may be compromising brain health. In contrast, the *Bifidobacteria* levels either remain the same or are elevated. Elemental diets should be performed with medical supervision; if you have brain-related symptoms and bloating, gas, and pain, particularly after a carbohydrate meal, I recommend you see a nutritionally oriented physician or licensed naturopathic physician. While not 100 percent accurate, the lactulose hydrogen breath test is a simple, noninvasive, and adequate test for SIBO. See the Appendix for more details.

An overgrowth of certain types of bacteria may also be contributing to obesity, according to some very interesting new studies from the Washington University School of Medicine. These researchers have found that obesity alters the makeup of the gut microflora, and when certain types of bacteria begin to dominate, there is enhanced uptake of calories from fibers and increased storage of energy into fat cells! It is intriguing stuff, and certainly means that all the studies where folks lost weight eating yogurt may have to be re-evaluated—could the beneficial bacteria in yogurt play a role in weight loss? It is entirely possible. A final word on SIBO: new research published in the *Asia Pacific Journal of Clinical Nutrition* (2004) shows that a diet low in omega-3 fatty acids encourages SIBO! Do you really need any more reasons to make sure you are getting enough omega-3 fatty acids?

Stress and Intestinal Bacteria

Psychological and physical stressors can have a considerable negative impact on your beneficial intestinal bacteria. In fact, you can think of stress as a potent antibiotic against the good *Lactobacilli* and *Bifidobacteria*. The first reports that stress could impact the intestinal flora came in the late 1970s, when researchers showed that states of anger and fear can increase potentially negative *Bacteroides* by almost tenfold. Following this, Russian researchers reported on studies they had been conducting with a group of cosmonauts who were preparing for flight. In the days leading up to the launch, as nervous-emotional stressors became higher, there were marked decreases in *Lactobacilli* and *Bifidobacteria*. It was the *Bifidobacteria* that appeared to be extremely vulnerable to preflight emotional stress. Even after the flight, the microflora remained altered, with increases in *Clostridia* species and long-term effects on beneficial bacteria. In addition to the preflight emotional stress, flight conditions, including restraint stress and physical demands, led to significant decreases in *Lactobacilli* and *Bifidobacteria*.

Endurance athletes are well known to have gastrointestinal complaints. In one study it was shown that in endurance athletes who train more than thirteen hours per week have lower levels of *Bifidobacteria*. The athletes who work to near exhaustion actually had a fecal microflora that was very similar in profile to chronic fatigue syndrome except for one glaring difference: about 60 percent of the athletes had very low levels of *Enterococci*. Remember *Enterococci*? It's the same bacterial group that in high numbers is associated with neurological, psychiatric, and cognitive dysfunction. It could be that *Enterococci* overgrowth in the gut is playing a role in brain and behavior. Experimental research shows that a decrease in *Bifidobacteria* and a rise in *Enterococci* is associated with chronic inflammation in the GI tract, and infants with allergies are more likely to have high levels of *Enterococci*. When animals are switched to a nonnatural, semisynthetic diet, they have lowered *Lactobacilli* and increased *Enterococci* and are more susceptible to experimental infections.

Some researchers have suggested that *Enterococci* might have toxic effects that, when in excess, compromise the intestinal barrier. As we discussed previously, a porous intestinal barrier allows unwanted materials, including toxins, to gain access to the inside. In contrast, probiotics such as *Lactobacillus plantarum* 299v protect the intestinal barrier and have been shown to prevent intestinal permeability induced by pathogenic (bad) bacteria. Experimental studies clearly demonstrate that *Lactobacilli* and *Bifidobacteria* can keep the growth of *Enterococci* in check.

Numerous reports from animal studies show that stress can alter the intestinal microflora. Overcrowding and excessive heat can increase *Enterococci* and decrease *Lactobacilli*. Noise stress and a feeling of being trapped will lower *Lactobacilli* in laboratory animals. Psychological stress encourages the growth of oral *Candida* in animals—an overgrowth that can be inhibited with the anti-anxiety medication Xanax. This is incredible research, especially when you consider that when *Candida* overgrows, it can compromise mental sharpness, lower mood, and increase anxiety and fatigue. Researchers showed that there were marked increases in *Candida* species in those who survived the devastating 1995 Hanshin-Awagi earthquake in Japan. Higher *Candida* levels were noted in subjects who lived closer to severe earthquake-damaged areas.

Among primates, maternal stress during pregnancy can result in a reduction of both *Lactobacilli* and *Bifidobacterium* concentrations. In the offspring, measures of infant independence are correlated with infant total anaerobes (*Enterococci* is an aerobe), *Lactobacilli,* and *Bifidobacteria.* In other words, infant animals (in this case primates much like us) with higher *Lactobacillus* and *Bifidobacteria* species were more independent and exploratory than those with low levels. Lower *Lactobacilli* levels have been specifically correlated with the display of stress-indicative behaviors in animals.

The reason for the stress and good-bacteria connection is not known for sure, but it may have do with changes in intestinal motility, or the direct effects of stress chemicals. Research published in the *World Journal of Gastroenterology* (2005) showed that psychological stress interferes with motility, causes overgrowth of indole-producing bacteria in the small intestine, lowers *Lactobacilli,* and, if you need more, makes the intestine more permeable to undesirable material. Whatever the cause may be, it is clear that the consumption of probiotic bacteria may be advisable during times of stress.

The Brain in the Gut

The human gut contains more than 100 million nerve cells, so in a manner of speaking the intestinal tract has its own brain. The GI tract is a meeting place for nerves, intestinal bacteria, and immune cells. The bacteria themselves may influence the immune and nervous system by the manufacture of mood- and behavior-regulating neurochemicals such as sedating gamma amino butyric acids (GABA), serotonin, and other biologically active chemicals. Some incredible animal studies show that GI microorganisms can directly activate the nervous system, even in the total absence of a detectable immune response. Take the bacteria *Campylobacter jejuni* for example; we know that if we ingest a lot of them, we get really sick. But what are the effects of just a few of them? Oral administration of *Campylobacter jejuni* in tiny doses—not even high enough for the immune system to respond—caused mice to become fearful and less exploratory. Taking it further, the researchers found that even tiny amounts of oral *C. jejuni* can activate areas of the brain that govern information processing related to emotional and behavioral responses. So, it is entirely possible that unwanted bacteria in the GI tract might induce anxiety, depression, or other behavioral disorders without causing you to actually feel sick.

Final Thoughts

Every month, new studies come out and add a piece to the puzzle. The goings-on inside the gut can have profound effects on the brain, and ultimately on behavior. There is no question that stress is a big player here, but the old referral to the psychiatrist with the comment that it's "all in your head" is unlikely to encourage appropriate stress management. It only serves to make patients feel powerless or to blame themselves. Understanding how stress promotes a decline in beneficial bacteria and an increase in chronic inflammation is more likely to effect changes in lifestyle habits. We will talk more on that in the next chapter.

Now that we know that low-level chronic inflammation is involved in IBS, it provides an explanation for the mixed bag of brain-related symptoms that accompany the syndrome. For example, up to 90 percent of IBS patients have diagnosable major depression and/or an anxiety disorder. Inflammation can affect the cytokines, which alter mood, and can increase the opening of the blood-brain barrier.

Yes, inflammation in the gut has been shown in a number of studies to alter the permeability of the perimeter fence of the brain. Gut inflammation leads to alterations in sleep-wake, or circadian, rhythms, which in turn might account for some of the symptoms of depression, fatigue, anxiety, and increased chemical sensitivity that are common to IBS. Researchers from the United Kingdom have suggested that chronic, low-grade inflammation in the intestinal tract is a major player in a neurodegenerative disease that resembles Parkinson's disease. The widespread effect of low-grade inflammation in the gut clearly deserves more attention.

Interestingly, the brain cell–protecting spice turmeric has been shown to be very helpful in IBS. As previously discussed, turmeric is a

• • • CASE REPORT • • •

Jane is a thirty-one-year-old sales manager. She had a history of gastroin-testinal complaints, including constipation (alternating with occasional diarrhea), abdominal pain, bloating, and gas. She was recently diagnosed with irritable bowel syndrome (IBS). In addition, Jane reported mild anx-iety and depressive symptoms along with fatigue and a loss of mental clarity.

Quite often, the emotional symptoms are a byproduct of dealing with IBS, being on edge about when the symptoms are going to flare up—during travel, during a meeting at work, or at an entertainment venue, for example. Where is the nearest bathroom? Most IBS patients know that stress can worsen an already stressful medical condition. Mind-body med-icine and use of the relaxation response is an essential component in keeping IBS in check.

Jane had experimented with different foods and was certain that wheat and dairy were players in provoking symptoms. Emerging research from St. George's Hospital Medical School in London substantiates her experiences. Still, even with these foods restricted and use of mind-body techniques to keep stress in check, the symptoms would still occur, albeit to a lesser degree.

I had been following the progress of Irish researchers who were exam-ining a special probiotic for IBS. After a number of well-designed clinical trials, it was shown that the beneficial bacteria *Bifidobacterium infantis* 35624 could provide symptom relief to those with IBS when compared to placebo. This strain of *Bifidobacteria* improved bowel movements and reduced abdominal pain, discomfort, bloating, and distention. In 2005, *Bifidobacterium infantis* 35624 became commercially available in the form of a supplement called Align™.

Jane began taking Align™ on a daily basis, and within three weeks she experienced massive improvements that have continued while on the probiotic.

potent anti-inflammatory agent. Recently scientists showed that turmeric tablets dramatically improved the symptoms of those with IBS. Artichoke extract, a botanical known to promote the growth of beneficial bacteria, has also been shown to be helpful in reducing the symptoms of IBS. Probiotics, as you might expect, have also been shown to be of value in IBS and other gastrointestinal disorders. Certain strains of *Lactobacilli* and *Bifidobacteria* have been shown to down-regulate the production of inflammatory cytokines in IBS. In addition to this, a combination of pro-biotic cultures and multivitamin/mineral formula has been shown to improve depressive symptoms in a group of fatigued adults under stress. The study, published in the journal *Advances in Therapy* (2002), also showed that the mixture decreased the frequency of infections over six months by 29 percent and "gastrointestinal discomforts" were reported to be improved by 91 percent. I would really like to see this preliminary work followed up in a placebo-controlled study with just the probiotic.

The intestinal microflora in patients with autism may also be a key factor in the progression, or perhaps even the onset of the illness. Research published in the journals *Clinical Infectious Diseases* (2002) and *Applied and Environmental Microbiology* (2004) showed that children with autism have much higher levels of *Clostridium* bacterial species. This of course raises the notion that potentially toxic protein fermentation prod-ucts may have a negative impact on brain health in autism. In addition, the absence of a normal microflora might prevent proper detoxification of heavy metals and other chemicals implicated in autism and other brain-related conditions.

An elegant study by Dr. Martha Welch and colleagues from Columbia University in New York showed that chronic inflammation in the gut of animals can activate the same areas of the brain involved in autism (and I would add to that panic disorder, posttraumatic stress, and other psychiatric/neurological conditions). In particular, chronic gut inflammation activates the fear center of the brain called the amygdala, and its connections with other behavioral and stress-related centers. This is exciting work that supports the idea that the gut and the brain are more intricately tied than we ever imagined.

Summary

The autointoxication concept suggests that toxins produced in the human digestive system might contribute to disease. New scientific research validates this view. It is certainly not a reason to take laxatives or undergo potentially dangerous and time-wasting colonics. The emerging research suggests that the consumption of fiber and beneficial probiotic bacteria in yogurts and supplements may be the best way to promote normal bowel function. So-called friendly bacteria such as *Lactobacillus* and *Bifidobacteria* perform a host of functions to promote good health both locally in the gut and indirectly in the far reaches of the body. Beneficial bacteria have a beautiful working relationship with omega-3 fatty acids, and together they work in symbiotic fashion to promote health.

This influence of bacteria that reside or pass through the gut may be far greater than we ever dreamed of. Emerging research suggests that this influence includes brain health and even behavior. For now, we have more questions than answers, but as the pieces come together, the health of the gut should be a priority in all brain-related conditions . . . and it looks like the autointoxication theorists just might finally get some well-deserved recognition.

7

Dietary Context

I T NEVER CEASES TO AMAZE me when I think of how many popular weight-loss books overlook the lifestyle of the individual. Each and every eating experience occurs in an emotional and environmental context. For many who were fired up about high-fat, high-protein diets, there was little in the way of guidance about how to contextualize food. In fact, the obsession with counting carbs itself became a stressful way to eat—which is, as we will see, counterproductive. The Brain Diet plan is one that acknowledges that eating always occurs in context. Stress influences behavior and eating patterns, so stress management and consideration of lifestyle and the dietary environment are crucial when it comes to brain health. At the core of increasing the awareness of the dietary context is the discipline called mind-body medicine. We will have a close look at mind-body medicine and its ability to lower stress, and then we will examine how our thoughts and emotions can influence our dietary choices.

Stress and Its Consequences

The word *stress* gets thrown around quite a bit in our modern world, but what actually is stress, and what does it do for (or against) us? Stress can be defined as the thoughts, feelings, behaviors, and physiological changes that occur when the demands placed upon you exceed your perceived ability to cope. The stress-related thoughts, feelings, behaviors, and physical bodily changes are ultimately influenced by demands and perceptions. For example, some perceive heavy traffic as intolerable, and may use words like "I'm stuck," "I'll never get out of here," "there is no end to it," etc. Another individual might perceive traffic as part of the deal when living in or near a metropolis. That individual might use words like "delayed," "usual," or "temporary." Now if you throw a few extra stressors into the mix, such as having to go to the bathroom or being late for a meeting, obviously the demands grow higher and individual perceptions may change. Ultimately the person who wins in the game of stress coping is the person who actually believes he has some control over the situation. Neither party can change the fact that their bladder is full and the meeting started five minutes ago, but the stress-resistant person has coping skills and knows how to use stress-management techniques.

In chapter 4, Waist Management, we discussed the notion that potentially threatening saber-toothed tigers present themselves in many ways in our modern world. It has been reported that the average North American experiences about fifty brief stress-response episodes per day! The stress "response" is, of course, the automatic physiological changes and accompanying thoughts that occur in the event of a threat to our perceived safety. Even daily hassles or minor annoyances are enough to trigger measurable elevations in blood levels of the stress hormone cortisol. Perceiving some amount of stress is a good thing; it allows us to adapt to changes and perform at our best when we need to. However, huge problems arise when demands start to exceed perceptions too often and at a severe level. Both chronic, daily hassles and severe acute psychological trauma can wreak havoc on long-term health. As you may recall from chapter 4, chronic elevations of the hormones released from stress can damage our brains and encourage the deposition of abdominal fat. Two well-publicized studies published in late 2004 show that there are long-term health consequences of stress. The first, by Dr. Neal Krause of the University of Michigan, showed that a more frequent experience of traumatic life events in early life is highly predictive of ill health over age sixty-five. The second, by Dr. Elissa Epel and colleagues from the University of California, San Francisco, showed that both the perception and the chronic nature of stress can cause cells to prematurely age and die. In this case, women with the highest levels of perceived stress had markers of cellular longevity that were equivalent to a decade or more of additional aging compared to the low-stress group. The researchers looked at telomeres, which are known to protect the genetic material in our cells. Telomeres are small caps that insulate the genetic material much like the plastic tips on the end of a shoelace. The telomere length is correlated to the potential lifespan of the cell, and shortening is associated with an increased risk of damage and death. In this groundbreaking study, chronic stress, and a higher degree of perceived stress, was clearly associated with shorter telomere length.

I bring up stress in this chapter because both acute and chronic stressors have the potential to influence your food choices, which in turn ultimately affects your brain health. While research shows that not everyone alters their eating habits under stress, the vast majority, more than 80 percent of us, do make changes. For some, it means drastic reductions in food intake, while for others it means significant elevations in caloric intake via foods high in sugar and saturated fat. Whatever dietary direction stress may take an individual, it is the high-quality, nutrient-dense foods that get left out. More than 70 percent of those who both under- and overeat report an increase in snacking on foods that can hardly be described as brain foods. The fats and sugars may provide a very brief palatable comfort. This is, of course, the worst scenario, because it is under times of stress that we rely upon quality nutrition to prevent its damaging effects. Researchers from the University of Washington were among the first to report a stress–food choice relationship. In an elegant 1990 study, published in the journal *Psychosomatic Medicine*, these researchers showed that employees changed their dietary habits at times of major work deadlines. Dietary intake of total calories, total fat, and percentage of calories from fat were significantly higher in periods before deadlines versus more quiescent periods. Any dietary plan, be it to lose weight or improve brain health, that ignores such research is clearly an incomplete one. Around the same time, French researchers reported that total caloric intake among high-school students increases during stressful exam periods versus subsequent non-examination days.

In 1998, Dr. Andrew Steptoe of the University of London, U.K., and his colleagues made headlines when they published a report in the *British Journal of Health Psychology* showing that annoying daily stressors and hassles can trigger unhealthy eating habits. Among the nurses and teachers enrolled in the study, there was a significant (37 percent) increase in fast-food consumption during high-stress periods. Men in particular turned to beef, lamb, and pork with a 45 percent increase during times of stress. The research also supported the notion that cheese and sweets are indeed comfort- or mood-driven foods.

In a 2003 study in *Health Psychology*, researchers found that among more than four thousand teens, greater self-reported stress levels were highly correlated with more fatty food intake and less fruit and vegetable consumption. In addition, the adolescents who reported greater stress were more likely to consume snacks (obviously not carrot sticks) and more likely to skip breakfast. Breakfast, as we will discuss later, is a key to lowering stress and promoting learning, particularly in children.

In a study presented at the North American Association for the Study of Obesity's Annual Scientific Meeting in Vancouver (2005), researchers from the University of Kansas showed that at the end of a six-month weight loss regimen, those who reported the highest levels of stress and depression were more likely to regain weight. Self-reported stress and depressive symptoms were associated with greater amounts of fat and total calories consumed when assessed at various points from nine to eighteen months later. These results add to the evidence that stress can influence unhealthy dietary choices and compromise the ability to maintain a lean body.

So-called "stress eaters" or "emotional eaters" are known to eat more during times of stress, both acute (e.g., exam) and chronic (e.g., occupation, daily grind), but the why is not completely understood. The consumption of sweet carbohydrate-rich and protein-poor foods can increase the amount of tryptophan (an amino acid) that gets to the brain. Tryptophan is a required component in the manufacture of the mood regulating neurotransmitter serotonin. Research does support this idea, as stress-prone individuals subjected to stress are protected from depressed mood and elevations in our old friend cortisol when they consume carbohydrate-rich/protein-poor lunches and dinners. Such is not the case with a protein-rich/carbohydrate-poor diet. Experimental studies show that low brain serotonin levels will enhance the appetite for carbohydrates while high levels of the stress hormone norepinephrine enhances the intake of carbohydrates. It is also possible that the very palatable nature of sweet and junk foods may lead to the release of mood-regulating opioids in the brain. It is probably a combination of both factors. Whatever the case may be, it appears that stress or emotional eaters are attempting to self-medicate. It also provides a reason why so many people informed me that they were moody on the low-carb diet that swept North America.

Overactivity of the stress branch of the nervous system, the sympathetic branch, is associated with overeating and changes in blood hormones, and even tryptophan lowering; this in turn, may keep the cycle vicious by driving the further consumption of high-calorie foods. Overactivity of the sympathetic (stress) branch, or an increase in sympathetic tone, as it is often called, impairs digestion and interferes with sleep. We know from the last chapter on the gut-brain connection that chronic stress and impaired digestion has the potential to impact our beneficial intestinal bacteria and toxin load.

The sleep connection is also worthy of discussion. The ability of stress to interfere with sleep has further ramifications when it comes to food choices and dietary intake. When it comes to sleep, North Americans are definitely in debt, and it is a deficit that has been building over the years. Children of all ages sleep between one and two hours less than what they require each night. Average sleep for the masses has decreased by 1.5 hours per night compared to a hundred years ago. More than one-third of Americans sleep fewer than six and a half hours per night, yet just a century ago, the average night's sleep was nine hours. While some have suggested that only four or five hours of sleep is required, usually citing some famous historical figure who hardly slept, research shows otherwise. Sleep deprivation studies have shown a negative impact on mood and brain performance. That in and of itself should be just cause to consider sleep to be a major lifestyle priority—but there is another reason that pertains to the diet. Sleep deprivation increases sympathetic tone and concentrations of the stress hormone cortisol. If this is the case, then wouldn't it follow that sleep deprivation would be associated with having an increased appetite and being overweight? The answer is yes.

Experimental research shows that animals who are sleep deprived and have access to high-calorie foods increase their food consumption by 250 percent! Sleep deprivation is also associated with decreased leptin levels in humans, the hormone that curbs appetite. Humans also have increased levels of a hormone called ghrelin when sleep deprived. In contrast to leptin, elevations in ghrelin promote appetite, hunger, and food intake. Sleep deprivation in humans can lead to weight gain in as short a time as one week. If sleep deprivation can influence chemicals related to stress, mood, and weight, then wouldn't it suggest that in large population studies, those who sleep less will weigh more? The answer is also yes.

Dr. Robert Verona and colleagues from the Eastern Virginia Medical School showed that in about one thousand adults aged 18 to 91, sleep time was positively related to having a healthier body weight. An increasing BMI, from normal, to overweight, to obese, was associated with a decrease in total sleep time. In separate studies, other researchers showed that in five hundred middle-aged men and women, sleeping fewer than six hours and remaining awake beyond midnight was associated with an increased likelihood of obesity. Children may be particularly sensitive to the effects of sleep deprivation. In a study presented at the North American Association for the Study of Obesity's Annual Scientific Meeting in Vancouver (2005), researchers from Harvard Medical School showed that longer sleep duration at two years old was associated with a lower risk of being overweight or having a high BMI at three years old. In a separate study of more than eight thousand young people, there was a three times greater risk of obesity in children who slept fewer than eight hours when compared to those who slept ten hours. The proportion of young adults who are sleeping more than eight hours a night has been cut in half between the years 1960 and 2002. During the same period, the proportion of young adults in the fewer than seven hours per night category has also more than doubled. More and more young adults are turning to sleep medications—from 2000 to 2004 there was a 200 percent increase in spending among 20- to 44-year-olds on sleep medications. Even the use of sleep medications among 10- to 19-year-olds has increased by 85 percent!

Consider that sleeping just two hours more total per week, or less than twenty minutes per day, was associated with difference in BMI of 10 points between patients in normal weight and overweight/obese groups. A one-hour per week deficiency in total sleep time is associated with an average BMI increase of 5.4. Over time, this could easily transport someone from normal into the overweight or obese categories.

I think you can see where I am going with this; chronic stress interferes with sleep, and sleep deprivation promotes alterations in mood and changes in caloric intake. Sleep deprivation may drive obesity, and in turn, the chemicals (free radicals, cytokines) associated with carrying excess weight may alter mood and brain health.

In the context of the Brain Diet plan, sleep deprivation takes on additional importance because lack of sleep drives inappropriate food choices. Dr. Karine Spiegel and colleagues from the University of Chicago have been looking at the relationship between food and obesity for a number of years. In a 2004 study in the *Annals of Internal Medicine*, they showed that not only does sleep restriction increase hunger, it was a driving force to consume more sweets, starchy foods, and other high-carbohydrate, high-calorie foods. Consumption of such foods increased by 33 to 45 percent in sleep-deprived individuals. In contrast, sleep deprivation had little effect on the appetite for fruits, vegetables, or high-protein nutrients.

There are some dietary supplements that may be helpful in sleep, including a type of milk protein called alpha-lactalbumin and some botanical remedies. These will be covered later on in the individualized treatment reviews. For now, we will move on to mind-body medicine, which is a medical discipline devoted to educating and empowering patients in the promotion of health.

Sleep Habits

Bedroom should be as dark as possible for maximum melatonin release.

Bedroom should be used for sleeping only. Remove the television and computer.

Bedroom environment should be organized and free of clutter, it should be an oasis from the rest of the world.

Bedroom temperature should comfortable—too much heat interferes with sleep.

Keep a regular schedule; go to bed at the same time, even on weekends.

Eliminate caffeine-containing beverages and food past 4 p.m.

Perform exercise in the daytime or early evening.

Alcohol should not be used as a sleep aid.

Avoid eating large meals late at night.

Go with warm milk and a small piece of whole grain toast.

Use relaxation techniques such as meditation in the evening.

Invest in a comfortable mattress.

Earplugs, soundproofing may help some, while others respond to steady a noise device (waterfall, ocean sounds, etc.).

Avoid TV news and action movies before bed—they can increase stress hormones, anxiety, and worry.

Mind-Body Medicine

The idea that mind and body are separate and distinct from each other has lingered in medicine for hundreds of years. This notion has been finally put to rest in recent years with the overwhelming research on the response to placebo used in clinical studies. More than 35 percent of subjects in clinical trials respond to the inert lookalike pill known as placebo. Often the pill of sugar can outperform the million-dollar chemical pill or natural product. The placebo response in digestive or intestinal disorders can reach almost 80 percent. In an editorial in the journal *Biological Psychiatry* (2000) by Dr. Irving Kirsch of the University of Connecticut, it was reported that between 65 and 80 percent of the response to antidepressant medication can be duplicated by placebos. His more recent review in the *British Medical Journal* (2005) indicates that the number may be even higher than 80 percent! Clearly, individuals who have a belief that they are taking a chemically active pill or herb can influence their own illness progression. This effect appears to be particularly strong in illnesses where there is a significant stress connection.

The placebo effect is often dismissed as a nontreatment, but is it really a nontreatment? I can't see how someone could make that argument when the sugar pill evokes such a positive effect on illness. New research shows that the placebo effect is not just an emotional response; University of Toronto researchers showed that the placebo response can actually change brain physiology. In their landmark study published in the *American Journal of Psychiatry* (2002), depressed patients who truly believed they were taking a powerful antidepressant but were actually taking a placebo had improvements in symptoms that were related to changes in brain glucose metabolism. A separate study that made waves in 2002 showed "sham" or simulated surgery was just as good for pain reduction as actual knee surgery for osteoarthritis.

The point is that there is a significant effect of the mind on the course of illness. These widely publicized studies certainly reinforce the connection, but they are hardly shocking to the researchers and clinicians of Harvard Medical School's Mind-Body Medical Institute, who have been examining the placebo effect for years. For clinicians and individuals who desire optimal health, the goal is to grab the thought processes and lessons of the placebo effect and utilize it, make it work for

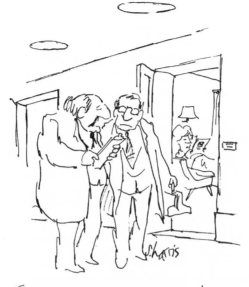

"FIND OUT WHO SET UP THIS EXPERIMENT. IT SEEMS THAT HALF OF THE PATIENTS WERE GIVEN A PLACEBO, AND THE OTHER HALF WERE GIVEN A DIFFERENT PLACEBO."

you in health promotion. Mind-body medicine is a broad term used for a number of techniques and therapies that take into full consideration that the mind (thoughts and emotions) can influence behavior and health status. Mind-body medicine also considers the influence of a disordered body on thoughts and emotions. The techniques of mind-body medicine include, but are not limited to: meditation, hypnotherapy, biofeedback, guided imagery and visualization, yoga, prayer, tai chi, breathing exercises, therapeutic writing and art, music and dance, and, perhaps most importantly, cognitive-behavioral therapy. There are more than two thousand studies in well-respected medical journals that give credibility to the value of mind-body medicine.

Meditation

The practice of meditation can be traced back more than three thousand years. In today's world, there are a host of different forms of meditation; however, there are two main categories that can be captured in general terms—mindfulness and concentration.

Mindfulness meditation is all about keeping yourself in the "here and now." It is the practice of paying attention to what you are experiencing in the current moment, without drifting off to the worry of the future or the experiences of the past. Mindfulness involves suspending judgment and letting go of opinions so that you will be less reactive. This fosters acceptance, self-reflection, and greater ability to handle difficulties without avoidance.

While the concept of mindfulness is not new—its value has been discussed for centuries in various traditions—only recently has the scientific world captured the health-promoting potential of mindfulness. As of 2005, there are well over one hundred citations related to mindfulness meditation in the scientific database Medline. Recent reviews of structured group programs called mindfulness-based stress reduction (MBSR) show that they are highly effective in lowering stress, decreasing anxiety, and lifting depression. In an eye-opening study published in *Psychosomatic Medicine* (2003), researchers showed that an eight-week mindfulness course was associated with greater activation of areas of the brain associated with positive mood. Even more wild was that those who shifted to a greater activation in this positive (happiness/optimism) area had a better immune response to the flu vaccine. These impressive results were not recorded on the day the eight-week program ended—the changes were documented between entry into the program and four months after its completion.

In a recent study of an eight-week MBSR program in nursing students, the results showed greater well-being and improved coping skills. The study, published in the *Journal of Nursing Education* (2004), showed that mindfulness decreases student anxiety and contributes to—get this—a decreased tendency to take on the negative emotions of others. That is something we could all use, but for nurses and other professions that see people not at their best, it's worth its weight in gold.

As beneficial as the actual MBSR programs are, and I encourage anyone with significant stress and/or a chronic illness to take advantage of one, it is important to note that even learned mindfulness from books, audio, etc., can be helpful. In a 2003 survey published in the *Journal of Personality and Social Psychology*, researchers showed that greater awareness and being mindful in life from day to day is correlated with enhanced well-being. Researchers from the University of Rochester found that among 1,500 adults surveyed, higher scores on a scale of mindfulness is associated with improved mood, optimism, life satisfaction, and willingness to attempt new experiences. Individuals were assessed on mindfulness using fifteen questions, including those related to focus in the present, preoccupation with past and future. One question in particular was directly related to a mindfulness-diet connection—"Do you snack without being aware that you are eating?" Answering yes to this question may be a sign to work on mindfulness. Forgetting someone's name two seconds after they have told you is another day-to-day example of the need for mindfulness.

Mindfulness meditation can be conducted while seated using meditative breathing, while doing yoga, or while walking in a slow and observant fashion. Meditative breathing is otherwise known as diaphragmatic breathing, where it is the abdomen, and not the upper chest, that moves in and out. Some suggest placing your hand over your belly button, feeling it move with your breaths, and imagining a balloon being inflated. You can think of the air flow in abdominal breathing as "in and down" as you develop a natural abdominal movement.

Many individuals react to stress by over-breathing, which in turn can restrict blood flow to the head and promote dizziness, anxiety, fatigue, and other bodily symptoms. For example, panic disorder is associated with a dysfunction of the area of the brain that controls respiration. Panic-prone individuals are very sensitive to carbon dioxide exposure and to hyperventilation. Highly consistent findings show a less stable respiratory pattern, even in relaxed states, in patients prone to panic attacks versus healthy controls. While not every person with panic attacks is sensitive to carbon dioxide and hyperventilation, many are, and research shows that breathing exercises and "retraining" the breath can relieve anxiety.

As far back as 1938, studies have shown that breathing retraining achieves a reduction of bodily complaints, anxiety levels, and frequency/intensity of anxiety attacks. Breathing exercises provide individuals with a sense of control in dealing with acute and chronic stress. Knowing that at any moment you can kick in to your meditative breathing teaches you that you can short-circuit the vicious cycle of stress hormones, physiological symptoms, and subsequent interpretation of danger.

In 2005, Japanese researchers showed that mindfulness may be associated with enhanced serotonin function in the brain. This is an important finding when you consider that serotonin depletion can worsen the irregularity of respiratory function, and that antidepressant medications that enhance serotonin may reduce the hyper-sensitivity to carbon dioxide in panic disorder. Dietary depletion of the amino acid tryptophan, which is required for serotonin production, leaves people with panic attacks more prone to a carbon dioxide–induced panic attack. Consistent, regular practice of mindfulness may raise the threshold of panic by altering brain chemistry.

Whatever its physiological mechanisms, there is no question that mindfulness meditation is a worthwhile venture when it comes to stress management and the reduction of anxiety and depression. Concentration meditation is somewhat different, but the beneficial end result remains the same—it's a matter of finding what works for you, or even using both on a regular basis. Concentration meditation infers that there is a focus of cognition—an object (e.g., picture or candle), a word/phrase/mantra, or visualized object. Concentration meditation removes focus away from all of the things that make our minds cluttered and stressed. The every-day hassles, worries, and aggravations are no longer prioritized in the stressful mind. While that in itself is a welcome break, the regular prac-tice of concentration meditation has physiological payoffs far greater than simply "relaxing." Research in the journal *Medical Science Monitor* (2004) showed that those who regularly practice meditation using a mantra had higher morning levels of serotonin and melatonin. The melatonin levels were 123 percent higher in the meditators than in the healthy controls. You are probably aware that melatonin is an important sleep hormone, antioxidant, and immune-regulating chemical. Low levels of melatonin have been associated with sleep difficulties, various cancers, depression, and chronic pain states such as fibromyalgia.

The benefits of the relaxation response can be directly observed and enhanced with the use of a brilliant new handheld biofeedback device called the StressEraser™. The device provides users with visual and clearly understandable feedback on biological and physiological changes that occur with breathing exercises and meditation. The StressEraser works on the finger pulse because the pulse rises and falls in a wavelike manner while reflecting the activity of the different nerves that control the stress and relaxation responses. The StressEraser displays your pulse rate waves in the middle of the screen and, via a few simple symbols, allows you to quickly determine which branch of the nervous system (stress or relax-ation) is in dominant mode. For more details, see the Appendix.

Perhaps the best known form of concentration meditation is the relaxation response developed by Dr. Herbert Benson of Harvard Medical School. After scientifically evaluating the physiological effects of transcendental meditation, Dr. Benson came to learn that focusing attention on a simple mental stimulus (word, phrase, image) brought about a reduction in sympathetic nervous system activity, lower heart rate, decreased muscle tension, lower blood pressure, and a respiratory rate in the complete opposite direction to hyperventilation. What he found was that just as there is a well-defined and automatic stress response, so too is there an opposing relaxation response that can be brought on by a form of meditation.

After years of scientific research, Dr. Benson determined that the relaxation response can be initiated by the following:

- A quiet, comfortable environment, with you in a comfortable position.
- Conscious relaxation of the muscles of the body.
- Repetition of a simple mental stimulus such as a word, phrase, image, or prayer.
- A passive mental attitude toward the process itself and any intrusive sounds or thoughts.
- Duration of ten to twenty minutes.

What we know about the relaxation response is that both the mind and body are calmed, which in turn can recondition the stress response to react more appropriately to stressors. The relaxation response reduces arousal in the emotional center of the brain called the limbic system. This in turn leads to a reduction of stress-related hormones such as epinephrine and cortisol. Of course, lower stress and lower cortisol may lead to a decreased storage of abdominal fat, lower stress, and more appropriate food choices.

The regular practice of the relaxation response can reduce overactivity of the stress branch of the nervous system, and over time, it can lower the threat level perceived by stress-prone individuals. Research published by Dr. Benson of Harvard, and colleagues from other universities from around the world, have shown that the relaxation response is helpful in many brain-related conditions, from migraines to irritable bowel syndrome. The effects of the relaxation response have been confirmed using sophisticated brain wave and MRI studies. The results show that the relaxation response can regulate brain waves associated with relaxed wakefulness, a state of maximal awareness, deep insights, and intuition.

Change Your Thinking

All of us could use a little cognitive-behavior therapy (CBT) once in a while. CBT is a great way to change the negative thinking that can compromise brain health. Negative thinking feeds the stress cycle and promotes poor lifestyle (behavioral) choices. CBT is well known to be helpful for anxiety, depression, and other chronic illnesses. CBT is not limited to very ill people; it can also be used as a means to promote and maintain health. Certain thoughts and beliefs related to the perception of stressors can have a negative effect not only brain function and mood, but also on dietary choices.

One goal of CBT is to identify and address negative thoughts and beliefs. Cognitive distortions, or so-called "faulty-thinking" patterns, are those that eliminate the positive, overexaggerate the negative, and invoke a lot of "what if?" type future-thinking. The thoughts are almost always "What if . . ." and a negative is tacked on to the end of the sentence. For example, "What if I do poorly on the test?" "What if I forget my lines?" "What if my presentation is not well received?" "What if that stomach ache is cancer?" "What if the elevator gets stuck?" and on and on it goes.

Beyond the negative "what if" phrases, stressed individuals then take it to the next catastrophic level; the failed test means that the individual will never get a decent job and will never be successful, the elevator that gets "stuck" will mean missing the meeting and losing the important business deal. Our "what ifs" usually feed into more catastrophic thinking, which, in turn, feed the stress chemicals. Remember, when you think it, you can start to believe it, and your body will respond as if the stress is actually happening.

More fuel on the stress fire comes from leaping to conclusions. Stress-prone individuals are Olympic athletes when it comes to the conclusion jump. In order to cut off the stress cycle, it is important not to draw firm conclusions before the facts are in. Reshaping thoughts and beliefs, underscoring the positive what ifs, and staying in the moment can minimize stress and enhance coping skills.

Most of the negatives addressed in CBT are related to self-talk. We walk around this earth having a constant inner dialogue. These thoughts influence our feelings, so it only stands to reason that positive self-talk will generate positive feelings. There are so many things in this world that we can't control, but the one thing that we *can* control is our self-talk. Thinking "I am competent and I can cope with this" is clearly a better option than "There is no way I can do this." Thinking "What if my presentation goes great?" is definitely better than "What if the presentation is too much for me to handle?" Thinking and believing that you are calm, in a relaxed state, and in control of your breathing is much more likely to give you a sense of control. Learning to use your control over self-talk will help to keep yourself in the here and now.

Mental Imagery

Part of past recollections and future thinking is the inclusion of imagery. Images are an essential component of human thought, and just like our self-talk, this can be both healthy and health-compromising. Stress-prone and anxious individuals often use mental imagery to play out worst case scenarios in their minds. Not meeting a deadline conjures up images of the boss saying, "Pack up your things!" These images, just like the negative self-talk, bring about stress-related physiological changes. If negative mental imagery can promote cortisol production and other stress changes, then wouldn't it seem plausible that positive imagery would do the opposite, and dampen down the sympathetic overdrive? Research shows that it can indeed do just that. There are numerous studies showing the benefits of mental imagery in lowering stress levels and decreasing anxiety. Guided imagery, as taught by mental health professionals, has been shown to be helpful in many brain-related medical conditions, including headaches, multiple sclerosis, fibromyalgia, and anxiety disorders.

Imagery has been found to be particularly well suited to hospital settings, where it is used as a means of pain management. Pleasant guided imagery often invokes the visualization of beautiful scenes of nature, perhaps a serene and quiet beach surrounded by green covered cliffs, or a waterfall in the midst of natural tropics. We have an amazing ability to capture these scenes in our minds, so why not take advantage of it to promote a healthy brain. There are numerous books, audio recordings, and

computer programs to provide guidance in using imagery and visualization. If it is beyond stress management and to be used to treat a brain-
related condition, I would recommend at least a couple of sessions with a
professional to get you started with mental imagery.

Music Therapy

Guided imagery goes really well with a side of music therapy. Music has been
used for centuries as a means to enhance mood and well-being. Music has
been used successfully in the treatment of brain related conditions, from
Alzheimer's and autism to social anxiety and schizophrenia. Researchers
from Case Western Reserve University and the Tzu-Chi General Hospital
in Taiwan found that sedative music selections, listened to for forty-five
minutes at bedtime, improves sleep duration and quality. There was also less
daytime sleepiness and cognitive dysfunction. A separate team of international researchers also showed that relaxing music (compared to silence) can
prevent sharp rises in cortisol after psychological stressors.

Different types of music mean different things to different people, but
some observations have been made regarding particular types of music.
For example, researchers from the Institute of HeartMath found that listening to fifteen minutes of grunge rock music increased hostility, sadness, tension, and fatigue. There were also reductions in caring,
relaxation, mental clarity, and vigor. The study included males and
females aged 12 to 76 years old, so one might imagine that the grunge
rock music would have a negative effect only on older adults. Yet, after
listening to the grunge music, even the teens reported significant
increases in stress-related emotions. In contrast, the researchers found
that so-called "designer music" (music designed/composed to produce
beneficial physiological/psychological effects) increased caring, relaxation, mental clarity, and vigor. The designer music, taken from the CD
called *Speed of Balance* by artist Doc Lew Childre, also decreased hostility, fatigue, sadness, and tension. Both New Age and classical music produced beneficial effects in some markers, including relaxation and
decreased tension, but neither matched the overall effects of specifically
designed music. Much like Dr. Benson uncovering the best way to induce
the relaxation response, researchers from the Institute of HeartMath are
uncovering the musical means to busting stress.

Yoga/Tai Chi

Yoga and tai chi bring together physical movement and the emotional being, a union of which is what mind-body medicine is all about. Among Westerners, Hatha yoga has become the most popular from of yoga. Hatha (physical) yoga incorporates specific movements and postures (*asana*) and breathing techniques (*pranayama*) that are often used along with meditation. In Hatha yoga, it is the breath that takes center stage; through proper breathing control, one can absorb the life-force, or *prana*. The breath is the essential component in the union of mind and body.

Research on Hatha and other forms of yoga has been growing steadily in recent years. Yoga has been shown to improve sleep and reduce the perception of stress. Researchers from Bangalore, India, showed that regular practice of yoga may be akin to a sleeping pill. In adults with insomnia, those practicing yoga reduced the time it takes to get to sleep down from forty minutes to ten minutes. Yoga practice also added an hour to total sleep time. In a separate study, published in the *Annals of Behavioral Medicine* (2004), researchers showed that Hatha yoga can reduce cortisol levels and improve scores on the Perceived Stress Scale.

Tai chi also combines physical movement, breathing, and meditation. As you might imagine, the end result of this combination is usually a more relaxed individual with a clear mind. Tai chi focuses on abdominal breathing in coordination with movement. The breathing and movement are said to enhance the flow of energy (*qi*, pronounced chee, and don't let anyone tell you otherwise) throughout the body. Research shows that regular practice of tai chi improves cardiovascular and lung function, strength, balance, flexibility, blood flow, and psychological parameters. As with yoga, tai chi has also been shown to reduce the stress hormone cortisol. An added bonus is that yoga has been linked with weight loss. The beneficial effect of yoga on keeping the weight off is not only due to it being a physical activity, it also works by way of its ability to help with mindfulness, including being mindful of signals related to fullness.

Exercise

Beyond yoga and tai chi, the research related to other forms of exercise in moderation on well-being is very solid. Dr. Kenneth Fox of the University of Bristol, U.K., stated in the journal *Public Health Nutrition* (1998) that moderate regular exercise should be considered as a viable means of treating depression and anxiety disorders and improving mental well-being in the general public. Since then, a wealth of research has supported his position. The bulk of the evidence is related to an elevation of mood and an antidote to depressive symptoms. However, in the mental-health realm, two new studies on exercise and its effects on anxiety are worth noting. The first, in the *American Journal of Psychiatry* (2005), showed that exercise has a direct, acute anti-panic effect. The background to this exercise study is the recent discovery that the injection of a brain chemical called cholecystokinin tetrapeptide (CCK-4) can induce panic attacks even in healthy adults who have never had a history of panic. Give enough CCK-4 and eventually most adults will experience the horrible feelings that those with panic disorder must endure. Amazingly, thirty minutes of aerobic exercise prior to the injection of CCK-4 significantly lowered panic scores versus simply having a quiet rest before the injection.

Also in 2005, researchers writing in the *International Journal of Emergency Mental Health* reported that a twelve-session aerobic exercise program was helpful in reducing at least some of the symptoms of posttraumatic stress disorder (PTSD). This is an important study because PTSD can linger for years, and while traditional drug and talk therapy are often effective in symptom management, a significant number of PTSD patients are not helped with these first-line approaches. Just to be clear, we are not talking about exhaustive exercise here—moderation is the key. Although intense exercise can generate free radicals, regular moderate exercise has been shown to enhance the body's innate ability to defend against oxidative stress—both in animals and humans.

HERMAN®   by Jim Unger

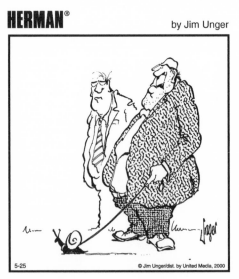

5-25   © Jim Unger/dist. by United Media, 2000

"He gets me out for a little exercise!"

A brain chemical called neuropeptide Y has been shown to be low in depression, and it has also been shown to be a marker of stress resilience. Experimental studies have recently shown that exercise enhances neuropeptide Y, and these increased levels are associated with new brain cell growth and an antidepressant effect. The benefits of exercise on mental health could easily make up an entire chapter. There is no need for me to go on and on about it. Against a background of animal studies showing that exercise activates proteins that are known to enhance brain cell survival and growth, consideration of two landmark human studies published in the *Journal of the American Medical Association* (September 2004) should speak volumes.

The first, by Dr. Jennifer Weuve and colleagues from Harvard, showed that physical activity, and walking in particular, is associated with significantly better cognitive function and the prevention of cognitive decline in older women. In the second study, Dr. Robert Abbott of the University of Virginia found a similar effect in males. Men who walked the least had an almost doubled risk of dementia compared to those who walked more than two miles per day.

Walking is great for brain health, and new research suggests that the effect may be enhanced by walking on an uneven surface. Cobblestone walking pathways are very popular in China, particularly in the urban centers of Beijing and Shanghai, where factories, hotels, and residential areas incorporate cobblestone paths for health promotion. The non-uniform surface of cobblestone paths encourages the activation of many muscles of the legs and ankles, muscles that are underutilized in our perfectly flat, manmade environment. Research shows that standing on a shifting, slightly uneven surface reduces fatigue, prevents the pooling of blood in the lower limbs, decreases the stress placed on the cardiovascular system, and keeps more blood up in the brain where it belongs.

In a separate study published in the *Journal of the American Geriatrics Society* (2005), walking on cobblestone mats for less than one hour three times a week produced notable health benefits in adults over sixty. Specifically, after sixteen weeks, there were significant improvements in balance and mobility as well as a valuable reduction in blood pressure. The control group walking on flat surfaces also improved, but not to the same degree. The good news is that you don't have to take a trip to China to walk on cobblestone paths—the long cobblestone mats used by the

Oregon Research Institute for the study are now commercially available. See the Appendix for details.

In contrast to what you might expect, exercise can actually decrease appetite for an hour or more. There is little evidence that humans over-consume calories after exercise; in fact, exercise appears to diminish the appeal for high-fat choices. Hopefully, researchers will examine the effect of exercise on dietary choices more closely. In the meantime, we know that it can maintain a healthy brain, help with waist management, lower stress, improve sleep, elevate mood, and diminish anxiety. In addition to the long-term effects of physical activity, there are immediate effects as well. Researchers from the University of Bristol in the U.K. showed that midday exercise can improve productivity, mental performance, and mood on days when workers are physically active. Aerobics, yoga, and stretching all decreased the expected afternoon fatigue. Remember too, that there is a relationship between dietary factors and exercise when it comes to weight loss. Dr. Peter Howe and colleagues from Australia high-lighted this connection when they showed that exercise plus fish oil helps to trim down the abdominal fat better than fish oil or exercise alone. So, eat your sardines, take your fish oil supplements, and start moving your feet.

Heart Rate Variability

If you haven't heard about the importance of heart rate variability (HRV), you will soon. HRV is becoming established as one of the most important ways to identify the health of the brain-heart connection and our resilience to stress. Simply put, you want your heart rate to be vari-able. The ability of the heart rate to elevate and decrease in response to breathing, stress, posture, hormones, and blood pressure is a marker of good health. Individuals with a decreased HRV are more likely to die from cardiovascular disease than those with normal or higher variability.

Chronic stress can compromise HRV and this, in turn, leaves the individual less able to respond appropriately to stressors. It is now becom-ing increasingly well known that having depression and/or an anxiety dis-order significantly increases the risk of dying from cardiovascular disease. Both depression and anxiety are associated with reduced HRV. The good news is that diet and lifestyle can positively influence HRV. In particular, exercise and omega-3 fatty acids have been shown to improve HRV. Other ways to improve HRV may also include intermittent fasting; decreased intake of saturated and omega-6 fats; decreased refined carbohydrates; and increased fruits, vegetables, and nuts. Mind-body techniques such as meditation have also been shown to improve HRV. Researchers from the Institute of HeartMath have published a number of studies showing that disengaging from negative mental and emotional reactions and shifting attention to the area of the heart while self-generating a positive feeling state (e.g., caring or appreciation), can improve HRV. Designer music may also play a role in assisting individuals to generate positive emotional states centered in the heart.

See Green

A number of published studies have suggested that the urban environment is a risk factor for mental illness. The strongest evidence comes from a study in the *British Journal of Psychiatry* (2004), in which researchers looked at the entire 4.4 million population of Swedish 25- to 64-year-olds! Incredibly, they found that the more urbanized the environment, the higher the rates of psychosis and depression. In fact, those living in the most urban environments were up to 77 percent more likely to experience psychosis, and up to 20 percent more likely to experience depression than rural dwellers. Of course, the urban environment can bring with it more daily hassles, noise, less social support, substance misuse, insufficient light, and tight living quarters. There is, however, the visual factor related to the urban environment—little greenery, and a lot of bricks, glass, and cement.

Dr. Frances Kuo and Andrea Taylor of the University of Illinois published an eye-opening study in the *American Journal of Public Health* (2004), which suggests that the effect of greenery cannot be overlooked. In a national study of attention-deficit hyperactivity disorder (ADHD), they found that outdoor activities conducted in green (natural) settings significantly reduced symptoms more than the same activities conducted in built outdoor (urban-style) and indoor settings. The age, gender, income, community type, or geographic region made no difference—only that the activity be conducted in a green, natural environment.

As proposed by environmental psychologist Dr. Stephen Kaplan, the reason we feel so refreshed after time spent in natural settings is that in nature there is little effort required to inhibit unwanted stimuli. In unnatural settings, such as sitting in front of a computer screen in an office or shopping in a crowded, colorful mall, there is a requirement to deliberately direct attention to the task at hand, and inhibit a multitude of unwanted stimuli. Seeing green appears to ground us from overload. Dr. Kuo and her colleagues, as well as other researchers, have shown that nature-based environments can improve cognition and reduce impulsive behavior. It doesn't mean you need to drive to the countryside, as the research shows that even green views can make a tremendous difference. However, the work of Dr. Kuo says a lot about why we get in our cars and head for the state, provincial, and national parks to recharge our batteries and de-stress.

Another reason to get outdoors and see some green, or even better, to put yourself into a forest environment, has to do with the exposure to negative ions in the air and the abundance of natural chemicals that are devoid in the air of urban environments. Days with high air pollution have been associated with a disproportionate number of psychiatric emergency calls, and as mentioned in chapter 5, the influence of unnatural environmental chemicals on mood, perceived stress, concentration, and cognitive functioning has been noted. Interestingly, higher air particulate matter has been associated with negative changes to heart rate variability and an increased risk of dying from cardiovascular disease.

Negative air ions are natural components of air and breath, which are depleted within polluted, enclosed, and air-conditioned rooms. Negative ions are also lowered by electronic devices, particularly those found in homes and offices such as computer screens and televisions. Negative air ions are known to influence mood in a generally positive way, and are much higher in natural settings, after rain, near oceans, waterfalls, and inside woodlands. According to research published in the journal *Indoor Air* (2004), negative air ions have been shown to promote our antioxidant defense system, lower blood lactate, and improve aerobic metabolism by enhancing blood flow. Research shows that small machines that generate negative air ions indoors are effective in treating seasonal affective disorder (SAD or the winter blues), and a recent study in the journal *Psychological Medicine* (2005) indicates that they can help lift nonseasonal depression as well. Research published in the *International*

Journal of Biometeorology (2005) shows that patients prone to panic attacks are much less likely to experience panic after rain when negative ion count is high.

Stick with a negative air ion device as used in the human research if you intend to buy one. The device used in the recent study comes from SphereOne Inc. See the Appendix for details.

In Japan, the practice of forest-air bathing is called shinrin-yoku, and it has been used medicinally for many years. In a study also published in the *International Journal of Biometeorology* (1998), researchers from the Hokkaido School of Medicine showed that walking in forest air lowers the stress hormone cortisol, decreases glycation (remember AGEs) of the red blood cells, and improves well-being. The effects of woodland walking appear to enhance the value of exercise alone. The authors attribute some of the benefits to the volatile compounds within the forest air. The interesting connections between mood, anxiety, and negative ions within natural settings deserve further research attention.

The Eating Environment

Multiple stimuli in the environment may not only lead to fatigue and cognitive overload, they may also make us eat more. Television is not a great way to go when it comes to improving brain function and providing a relaxed dining environment. As reviewed recently in *New Scientist* (July 9, 2005), children who watch the least TV between ages of five and eleven are most likely to be university grads, and children with a TV in their bedroom indeed watch more TV and have lower scores on standardized achievement tests. This suggests that TV is not educational in an academic way, and to make matters worse, it may encourage the consumption of anything but brain foods. In an interesting study published in the journal *Appetite* (2004), French researchers showed that adults eat more food when in the presence of engaging stimuli. Watching TV or listening to an audio detective story and eating at the same time caused a higher caloric consumption at meals. The stimulus appears to delay our awareness that we are full and that we should stop eating. If a TV can do that, just think about eating along with videogames!

In a study by Jennifer Utter and colleagues from the University of Minnesota, it was shown that high TV/video use was not associated with

healthier dietary choices among four thousand teenagers. TV/video viewing was actually associated with increased consumption of soft drinks,
fried foods, and snacks. Of course, every minute spent playing video
games and watching TV is one minute that a young child/teen is also not
being physically active. Separate research has shown that weekday TV
viewing is associated with more frequent visits to fast food establishments
among teens—and I don't need to tell you what goes on inside the doors
of fast food "restaurants"!

It has also been shown that more weekly TV viewing goes hand in
hand with a higher BMI and greater requests for commonly advertised
foods. In fact, almost 80 percent of food advertised to children during
those shows watched by youngsters is junk food, with sweets, candy, and
soft drinks accounting for 44 percent of the total. Clearly, it's not the sardine and salad companies that are advertising during young viewership
hours. This advertising is very effective too; in a study presented at the
North American Association for the Study of Obesity's Annual Scientific
Meeting in Vancouver (2005), researchers from the University of
Liverpool found that food advertisements increase children's preferences
for high-fat and high-carbohydrate foods. Children, it seems, have a
heightened awareness to food-related cues because they were able to
recall significantly more food ads versus toy ads.

When researchers from the Baylor College of Medicine followed
young three- to four-year-old children for three years, they found that
both physical activity and TV viewing could predict BMI. Time spent in
physical activity decreases BMI, and time spent watching TV makes it go
up. Interestingly, it was watching TV during the ages six and seven that
appeared to strongly predict a higher BMI. It is quite possible that this
sets the stage for later habits in life. Following this study, Belgian
researchers showed that on the average, just one hour of TV watching
equals the consumption of 156 calories. When you take away physical
activity, 156 calories per hour of TV over time can really add to the waistline and compromise brain health.

When it comes to videogames, half of the top sellers contain extreme
violence. Not only might such videogames prime the brain for violence,
as suggested in *New Scientist* (June 25, 2005) and in a large review published in the *Journal of Adolescence* (2004), they also significantly increase
stress. Consider also that violent videogames are not utilizing designer

music composed by Doc Lew Childre and the Institute of HeartMath. The soundtracks of violent videogames include techno and heavy metal music, which adds to the stress response. Dr. Sylvie Hebert and her colleagues from the University of Montreal showed that the techno music significantly increases cortisol levels in videogame players versus silent conditions. Despite what some have suggested, videogames are therefore not the way to go about smartening up the brain. Increased chronic stress, increased cortisol, connections to violence, decreased physical activity, associations with obesity, and overstimulation are not the attributes of brain-health therapeutics.

Scents of Relaxation and Clarity

The beneficial effects of certain aromas on the human psyche have been documented for centuries. Research on the effects of different scents on different people has a hundred-plus-year history, with a dramatic rise in interest over the last decade or so. The human olfactory system is intricately tied to our emotional control center, known as the limbic system. Even simply talking about an aroma can bring emotions and memories to the conscious level.

Essential oils are capable of reducing stress, promoting relaxation, and enhancing cognitive function—it all depends on the oil itself and personal preferences. For example, lavender may not be the oil of choice if you are getting ready to sit a final exam or give a career-boosting presentation. Dr. Mark Moss and colleagues from the United Kingdom published an elegant study in the *International Journal of Neuroscience* (2003). They showed that lavender actually diminished performance of working memory and attention-based tasks versus controls working in unscented cubicles. In contrast, those working in the rosemary-scented cubicles had significant improvements in performance related to memory factors. Both the lavender and rosemary groups reported higher levels of contentment versus controls. In a study recently published in the *International Journal of Psychophysiology* (2005), researchers from Coventry University, U.K., showed that peppermint oil can reduce daytime sleepiness versus a no-odor controlled condition.

Researchers from the Wheeling Jesuit University found that jasmine may promote sleep quality and increase alertness the following day. In a neat little experiment, they looked at the effects of jasmine, lavender, or no scent for three nights. The aromatherapy was infused into the rooms at such low levels that many were not even aware of any aroma at all. Not only did the jasmine sleepers toss and turn less frequently, they woke up feeling less anxiety the next day. The jasmine sleepers also performed better on cognitive testing the next day. Lavender was good too, but it couldn't match jasmine.

The same group from Wheeling recently showed that peppermint and cinnamon aromatherapy might quell road rage. They showed that prolonged driving led to the expected increased anger, fatigue, and physical demand, as well as decreased energy. Peppermint and cinnamon both decreased driving frustration and increased alertness while driving, and interestingly, the aroma of fast food made things worse! Peppermint was specifically shown to lower levels of anxiety related to the extended driving experience.

A low level of aromatherapy may be the best way to go, according to Japanese researchers from Kyoto University. They found that low levels of jasmine aroma could improve heart rate variability by dampening down the sympathetic nervous system. When it comes to an intense, high-level odor, then it all depends on whether you like the smell of jasmine or not. In those who told the researchers up front that they did not like jasmine, they had an increase in the activity of stress branch (sympathetic) of the nervous system when exposed to high levels of jasmine odor.

Yuka Saeki of the Nagano College of Nursing in Japan has also shown that aromatherapy may improve heart rate variability. In this case it was lavender in a warm foot bath that seemed to maintain parasympathetic activity for a longer period versus just the foot bath alone. Although I should point out that the warm foot bath was found to enhance the stress-dampening branch (parasympathetic) activity also, it was just not as long-lasting as that with lavender oil. Finally, a number of studies, including one recently published by researchers from the Konju National University in Korea, have shown that lavender aromatherapy can reduce aggressive behavior in those with dementia.

Hopefully further research will advance aromatherapy from folklore and retail beauty chains to credible therapeutic interventions. The incredible relationship between the olfactory system and the emotional center of the brain is ripe for further exploration. Given that many with brain-related conditions, from Alzheimer's disease to migraine headaches, from depression to seasonal affective disorder, have abnormalities in smell sensitivity, the plot thickens even more. For now, while we await more research, personally desirable and high-quality essential oils can be used for stress management.

Sauna

Heat-based therapy has been used as a means to relax, cleanse, and purify the body for thousands of years. It was the Finns who popularized sauna use in modern times, and the traditional steam-based sauna remains popular in health clubs today. Sauna would largely remain in the realm of health folklore if it were not for the efforts of researchers from Kagoshima University in Japan. They have published a number of studies showing that repeated sauna therapy improves cardiac function. These scientists have been examining a modern far-infrared-ray sauna. Infrared heaters warm the body in the same way as natural sunlight, using a wavelength of the light spectrum of the sun. Infrared is not to be confused with the dangerous ultraviolet spectrum of solar radiation.

The Japanese researchers, led by Dr. Akinori Masuda, showed in 2004 that far-infrared sauna can not only lower blood pressure, it can also lower oxidative stress. So not only is the sauna psychologically relaxing, we now know that it is quenching free radicals. The sauna was used for fifteen minutes a day, at 60°C, for two weeks. In a 2005 study published in the *Journal of Psychosomatic Research*, the same group showed that the once-per-day sauna for thirty-five sessions improved the fatigue, pain, sleep disturbance, and low-grade fever of chronic fatigue syndrome. It is fortunate that the Japanese researchers chose to work with far-infrared saunas because these units are now commercially available, compact, and easy to set up. Far-infrared saunas are well suited for home use, and many are made with CD players so you can relax to your favorite meditation tracks or designer music. See the Appendix for details.

Writing/Journaling

Research shows that confronting difficult life experiences thorough writing and art can have very positive effects on both emotional and physical well-being. When it comes to serious traumatic events, the writing and artwork would be best conducted with guidance from a mental health professional. There are more than a dozen studies showing that writing about stressful or traumatic events can improve various health conditions. Dr. James Pennebaker of Southern Methodist University and his colleagues have shown that writing about traumatic events can lead to subsequent (not immediate) improved mood and decreased use of health-care services. Taking advantage of therapeutic writing involves expression of your deepest emotions, including what you feel and why you feel it. Although you may want to share your writings, it is best to write as if it is just for you; this way you will be less likely to hold back. If events are constantly on your mind, it may be time to write things down or draw them out.

The 3 Cs

Dr. Suzanne Kobasa of the City University of New York identified three defining, and consistent, characteristics of so-called "stress-hardiness." Stress-hardy individuals have been found to embrace the 3 Cs into their worldview: Challenge, Control, and Commitment. They view change as a challenge and not something to be feared. Change is viewed as normal and is interpreted as a stimulus for growth and maturity rather than a threat. With regard to control, hardy personalities believe their actions do make a difference. They believe that they do have control and they are not merely victims of fate. In most cases, stress-hardy individuals in fact don't have more control over events than those who are stress-prone . . . they just believe they do. Finally, stress hardy individuals are immersed in what they do in life. They are committed to the end, and truly engaged in life.

Additional Notes

There are lots of other ways to keep stress in check. A full exploration of all the ways and means to manage stress is beyond the scope of this book. Other general considerations include, but are not limited to, organizational skills, time management, prioritizing tasks and life goals, delegating, letting go of procrastination, using humor, being optimistic, taking advantage of social support, and getting proper sleep. It is also important to appreciate recreation and take time out for yourself. Step out of the office and take ten or fifteen minutes for yourself—and ten or fifteen minutes away from computer screens and photocopy machines, known free radical generators. Surfing the Web might be fun for a few minutes, but new research shows that extended periods at visual display terminals (monitors) cause mental fatigue and increase both oxidative and psychological stress. Remember that the air surrounding computers is devoid of negative ions.

Take a break, limit your computer use, and turn off your cell phone once in a while—research shows that mobile phones blur the boundaries between home and work. It used to be that co-workers would only call others at home if it was really, really important—not so with the cell phone. For many, that little device means work never stops. Research in the *Journal of Marriage and Family* (2005) shows that cell phone use is linked to heightened psychological distress and reduced family satisfaction. Cell phones cause work to spill over into the home, and when that happens the result is not good for the worker and those around him or her. According to a study in the *Journal of Occupational Health Psychology* (2005), employees who take home their work with them feel more exhausted and irritable when they are at home.

Summary

Most popular diet plans provide little to no guidance on the dietary context. Considering the research that stress can drive dietary choices, it has always surprised me that stress management has been ignored by most nutrition authors. Nutritional intake always takes place in the context of lifestyle and environment. Both acute and chronic stress have the potential to influence the food and drink we put into our bodies. Research shows that about 80 percent of us make dietary changes under stress. The foods consumed in stress-related eating are far from healthy. Most stress eaters choose high-fat, high-sugar foods, and snacking is elevated. Stress drives fast-food selections and steers eaters away from fruits and vegetables. Choosing sugary carbohydrates and fatty foods may be a way to self-medicate by enhancing mood-regulating brain chemical production.

Chronic stress also interferes with sleep, and sleep deprivation promotes alterations in mood and ultimately promotes greater calorie intake . . . and so it goes. To manage stress, and short circuit the stress-driven consumption of non-desirable foods, we can take advantage of mind-body medicine. Thousands of published studies have shown that the human mind and body are far from separate. The placebo effect is the most obvious example of just how powerful belief can be on human health and physiology.

Mind-body medicine is a virtual buffet of techniques and therapies that consider the influence of the thoughts and emotions of the mind and their influence on the body. The relaxation response uncovered by Dr. Herbert Benson of Harvard Medical School is a well-established means to keep stress in check. Mindfulness meditation, yoga, tai chi, music, therapeutic writing, cognitive restructuring, visualization, and exercise can all contribute to the management of stress. Aromatherapy and sauna may also contribute to the benefits of established stress management and mind-body techniques.

Stress is ultimately about perception. Mind-body medicine and other stress management interventions can be "grounding," keeping the individual in the moment and away from the worries of the future and the negativity of the past. Mind-body medicine can improve coping skills, change perceptions, and recondition an unhealthy stress response.

8

Dietary Supplements

The use of nutritional and herbal products by North Americans has skyrocketed in the last decade. When I was a kid, chewable cartoon multivitamins and adult one-a-day multivitamin formulas were the only game in town. Today, Americans spend more than 15 billion dollars on dietary supplements, and we have gone from a couple of multivitamins to more than twenty-nine thousand commercially available herbal remedies and supplements. Studies consistently report that more than 40 percent of Americans and Canadians take at least one supplement or natural health product on a regular basis. The term natural health product encompasses vitamins, minerals, herbals, homeopathic remedies, Chinese medicines, Ayurvedic, Native North American remedies and various animal and plant products. North Americans generally use dietary supplements for three main reasons—to enhance dietary quality, as a preventative influence against disease, and as a "natural" means to address health problems.

Traditionally, those against supplements have been from the "you get everything you need from a healthy diet" camp, and those who support at least a multivitamin are from the "reality of the North American diet" camp. Obviously, I am in the latter camp; I don't discount the goal of a highly nutritious and complete dietary plan, it is just that most North Americans rarely achieve it. The facts are that we are not meeting the recommendations of the American USDA pyramid or Canada's Food Guide to Healthy Eating. A host of studies have shown that North Americans fall short; only 9 percent of young children (average age 9.9 years) meet the recommended number of servings from each group, and it is even worse for women of middle age and older—only 5.9 percent adhere to the pyramid. In a landmark Canadian study, researchers from McGill University found that the only group that met the recommendations of Health Canada for food group intakes were males aged 13 to 34. In 2002, a survey conducted by the *Globe and Mail* and Canadian Television showed that only one Canadian in six eats the recommended servings of fruits and vegetables. Only one in twenty meets the grain requirements. Yet amazingly, only 22 percent felt that there was room for improvement to their diet. Obviously this leaves millions of North Americans with subpar nutritional intake—and it leaves me at a loss as to why some dietetic professionals continue to live with their heads in the sand.

Another legitimate consideration is the research in both the United States and Canada showing that the vitamin and mineral content of fruits, vegetables, and meats has declined dramatically in the last half

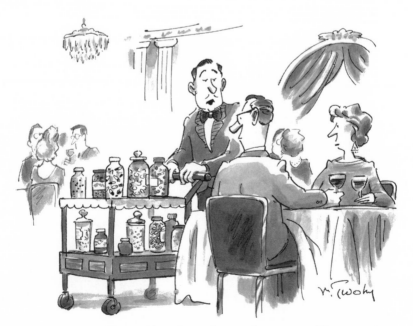

"Something from the supplement cart?"

century. Research published in the journal *Nutrition and Health* (2003) shows significant losses in magnesium, calcium, zinc, iron, and copper have been noted in the U.S. fruit and vegetable supply over the last half century. Canadian research (*Globe and Mail*, July 6, 2002) shows that almost 80 percent of fruits and vegetables tested showed drops in calcium and iron, 75 percent had decreased vitamin A, 50 percent had decreased vitamin C and riboflavin, 33 percent loss of thiamine, and 12 percent loss of niacin. A study published in the *British Food Journal* (1997) shows that the same phenomenon is occurring in the United Kingdom. In that study, all minerals in fruits and vegetables, with the exception of phosphorus, were significantly reduced over the previous fifty years.

All this doesn't mean we should stop educational efforts, nor does it mean that essential nutrients in supplement form can displace foods. The word *supplement* should be taken literally—it is an add-on to the best of dietary intentions. They are not called dietary substitutes, but rather dietary supplements—they will never be a substitute for a healthy diet.

At least the debate on taking a multivitamin on a daily basis is over. In a 2002 review of the evidence and accompanying editorial in the *Journal of the American Medical Association*, Harvard researchers recommended that all North Americans take a multivitamin formula every day. They made this suggestion because the potential protection against chronic illness clearly outweighs the minimal cost. They also concluded that there are no known health risks to taking the levels of nutrients as found in most multivitamin formulas. As quoted from Harvard's School of Public Health Web site, a daily multivitamin is "the least expensive insurance policy you can buy."

The conventional wisdom is that any old multi will do, but some patients with brain-related conditions and sensitivities may want to check the ingredient label first. Believe it or not, there are multivitamin/mineral preparations with commercial food dyes such as FD&C yellow #6 aluminum lake, and other additives. Patients with ADHD, chronic fatigue syndrome, fibromyalgia, and migraine headaches may be sensitive to such artificial ingredients. A good multivitamin and mineral formula should provide adequate levels of nutrients, and yet at the same time avoid unnecessary and potentially toxic "megadoses" of vitamins and minerals. Due to the bulky size of calcium and magnesium, these are not provided by most multivitamin/mineral formulas at adequate levels.

Additional supplementation of these nutrients for bone health should be considered.

While a daily multivitamin and mineral formula is a worthwhile health investment throughout life, perhaps the most critical time is during pregnancy and in early life. When it comes to intelligence and behavior, there is no question that genetics, stressors, and nutrition can play a role. The mold for IQ and behavior is set early on, inside the womb and in the first few years of life. That is not to say that experience, stress, and genetic and nutritional influences are nonexistent later on; of course they are there, but what happens nutritionally from conception to around age three can have tremendous repercussions for the next eighty-plus years. Research shows that nutritional inadequacy during pregnancy more than doubles the risk of having a male child who develops antisocial personality disorder in adulthood. Just in case you are unfamiliar with antisocial personality disorder, these are individuals who have no regard for the rules of society; they do bad things to people, animals, and property. Similar findings have shown that malnutrition during pregnancy increases the risk of serious forms of mental illness, such as schizophrenia or psychotic episodes, in the children.

In an incredible study published in the *American Journal of Psychiatry* (2004), researchers from the University of Southern California showed that malnutrition signs at three years old predicted more aggressive and hyperactive behavior at age eight. In addition, children with signs of nutritional deficiencies (cracking in the lips and corners of the mouth, hair dyspigmentation, sparse or thin hair, anemia) at age three were more likely to display externalizing behavior at age eleven and conduct disorder at age seventeen. Externalizing behavior and conduct disorder include chronic aggression, impulsivity, and destructive and oppositional behavior. Those with signs of malnutrition at age three were also the ones with the lowest IQ. As the authors suggest, it is entirely possible that malnutrition predisposes to neurocognitive difficulties, which in turn leads to behavioral problems in childhood and beyond. In the presence of genetics, stressors, and the environment, nutritional inadequacies can alter how a young person sees the world. The young brain is like a sponge, soaking up everything and laying down connections that last a lifetime. Without the full range of nutrients, the brain areas that take care of emotion and impulsivity may become disturbed.

But isn't malnutrition a thing of the past? Aren't all pregnant women taking steps to eat healthfully and take a daily multivitamin to ensure intake of much-needed folic acid? The answer is no. As per our discussions in chapter 7, stress drives food choices at all times, including pregnancy. While pregnant women who are more fatigued, stressed, and anxious actually eat more, it's the vitamins and minerals that they may fall short on. Dr. Kristen Hurley and colleagues from Johns Hopkins University found that stress in pregnancy is associated with higher intakes of breads and foods from the fats, oils, sweets, and snacks group of the food pyramid. Anxiety was also associated with higher intakes of foods from the fat, sweets, and snacks group. The moms-to-be who report stress and anxiety add more fuel to the genetic fire by consuming more calorie-dense but nutrient-poor foods. Consider that maternal stress and anxiety during pregnancy has been linked to subsequent hyperactivity, attention deficits, emotional problems, Tourette's syndrome, schizophrenia, depression, and drug abuse in offspring. While bathing the fetal brain in stress hormones that pass through the placenta may be the main culprit, the stress-induced changes to the maternal diet only compound the situation.

In the first few chapters of this book, we discussed the sad state of North American nutrition, and there is no evidence to show that unhealthy eating habits change to any large degree during pregnancy. Despite all the educational efforts on the benefits of taking a folic-acid-containing vitamin pill in order to prevent brain defects in the developing fetus, only 40 percent of women of childbearing age were taking a folic acid supplement in 2004. The message on the value of a folic acid supplement before and during early pregnancy is almost fifteen years old; it is a message that gets clouded when dietetic professionals maintain the old adage of "you get it all from your food." A simple daily multivitamin and mineral formula has the potential to change the child's future on this planet.

The first indications that vitamin intake during pregnancy might influence the IQ of offspring were published in 1956. Dr. Ruth Harrell and colleagues from Old Dominion University found that vitamin supplements (versus placebo) given to women during pregnancy and lactation produced higher IQ scores in their children three to four years later. The effect appeared to be due to the multivitamin filling in the nutritional holes in the background diet of the more urban pregnant women. The same beneficial effects were not evident in a group of rural dwellers who reared their own livestock and cultivated their own fruits and vegetables. A separate study in 1960 showed that only in those with low blood levels of vitamin C could orange juice significantly raise IQ scores when consumed regularly for six months. If you already had adequate blood levels of vitamin C, orange juice didn't make a difference.

There were six other older studies, published through 1984, that indicated that minor nutrients might play a major role in the IQ of children. Around the same time, Richard Lynn of the University of Ulster, Northern Ireland, was making world headlines as he demonstrated that the Japanese and other Asian groups have higher IQ scores than those in the Western world. Other investigators were reporting the same phenomenon, i.e., that Japanese students consistently outperform their Western counterparts in academic achievements. There are a number of reasons that may account for this, including genetics, school environment, and cultural influences. In an interesting study published in *The Journal of Social Psychology* (1992), researchers discovered that IQ differences between Japanese and North American children are evident before schooling even begins. Japanese kindergarten and first-grade children outperformed their Canadian counterparts on the Canadian Cognitive Abilities test on each battery—verbal, quantitative, and nonverbal. In 1989 Dr. Lynn proposed that nutrition was exerting a significant influence on intelligence. The scientific evidence so far has proved him right.

Genetics have turned out not to be the whole story. Inheritance accounts for only about half of IQ variability. The Japanese diet, at least until the recent Western fast-food influences, is one rich in colorful variety and deep in marine, brain-friendly, fats. In addition to the high omega-3 intake, the Japanese are quite fond of seaweed or sea vegetables. Most forms of seaweed are good sources of iodine and, as it turns out, research shows that low maternal iodine intake during pregnancy appears to set the table for ADHD and lower IQ by almost twenty points.

In separate research from the National Institute of Environmental Health Sciences, Dr. Julie Daniels and her team showed that maternal fish (non-contaminated) intake during pregnancy, and by infants post-natally, is associated with higher average developmental scores. Other researchers have found that omega-3 fatty acids supplemented during pregnancy and lactation enhanced the child's IQ when tested four years later. When Dr. Ingrid Helland and colleagues broke down the data in the journal *Pediatrics* (2003), they found that maternal DHA intake during pregnancy was the only variable of statistical significance for the children's mental processing scores at four years of age.

While IQ tests might be controversial—and they certainly have their flaws—intelligence has emerged as the best predictor of scholastic achievement. Academic success often translates into greater opportunity to choose employment of one's choice, financial rewards, etc. The research consistently connecting poor cognitive abilities and behavioral disturbances, which in turn are influenced by nutrition, has enormous implications for society. Based on the incredible research of Dr. Joseph Hibbeln of the National Institutes of Health, it may even be a matter of life and violent death. It was Hibbeln who identified the international relationships between lower omega-3 intake and higher rates of various depressive disorders. In 2001, he published a study that connected dietary omega-3 with the most extreme form of violence, homicide. What!? Yes, he showed that greater intakes of seafood rich in EPA and DHA correlated (very significantly) with lower rates of death by homicide in thirty-six nations examined. It seems outlandish, but it fits right in with other studies showing that lower levels of EPA and DHA are associated with increased hostile behavior in almost four thousand young adults in urban American cities, and also among aggressive cocaine addicts and violent prisoners.

Dr. Hibbeln and his colleague Dr. Norman Salem Jr. had been suggesting, as far back as 1995, that the massive increase in omega-6 linoleic acid was playing a role in the rise in violence in the twentieth century. In 2004, Dr. Hibbeln and his team showed that human consumption of linoleic acid–rich oils (omega-6) from 1961 to 2000 was associated with increased death by homicide in the United States, Canada, Argentina, Australia, and the United Kingdom. This, of course, does not prove causation, but when you add it to the existing research, particularly that related to omega-3 promoting IQ and diminishing the stress response, it certainly adds to the evidence.

Around the time that Dr. Lynn was proposing that diet can influence IQ, Dr. David Benton of the University of Swansea, U.K., published a study in the prestigious journal *Lancet* that rocked the nutrition world.

He and his colleague Gwilym Roberts showed that a basic multivitamin/mineral supplement given to thirty children improved IQ scores versus those taking placebo and those taking no pills at all. That average twelve- and thirteen-year-olds, who according to popular wisdom were well fed and nourished, could respond to a multivitamin pill was too much for old-school nutritionists. Some responded by quoting data that average British schoolchildren were meeting the recommended dietary allowance for vitamins and minerals. However, upon further review, there were pockets of children who were meeting less than 70 percent or even less than 50 percent of the RDA of many nutrients. The average RDA, as Dr. Benton has pointed out, is a statistic that says nothing about the individual. It also reflects minimal standards to offset disease and says little about optimal nutrition.

The Benton study was not a sign that we can build super-geniuses by providing multivitamins to children, it simply demonstrated that maybe young children are not as well nourished as we assume, and that complete nutrition deserved further research attention in relation to brain functioning. There were follow-up studies.

Since the now famous Benton and Roberts study, there have been twelve additional studies investigating vitamin and/or mineral supplementation on childhood intelligence. Nine out of the twelve studies showed a beneficial effect in nonverbal test scores with nutritional supplementation. As Dr. Stephen Schoenthaler of California State University showed in a number of his studies, children with mild nutritional deficiencies have the most to gain from multivitamin/mineral supplementation.

So, we know that adequate vitamin, mineral, and essential fatty acids intake is critical in maximizing brain function and IQ (one could also speculate fiber and dietary phytochemicals), and compromised IQ and brain dysfunction can set the stage for violent and impulsive acts. Wouldn't it then seem reasonable that proper nutrition and perhaps a multivitamin/mineral and/or a fish oil supplement might influence behavior in individuals prone to violence? Dr. Stephen Schoenthaler has shown that this is indeed the case. He has consistently shown for the last twenty years that when the nutrition of adult and juvenile inmates is improved, violent acts and antisocial behavior declines. In a 1997 study published in the *Journal of Nutritional and Environmental Medicine*, his team found that taking a daily multivitamin/mineral formula (versus placebo) reduced rule infractions by an average of almost 30 percent. Twenty-six of the subjects had blood levels checked for nutritional status; in those who recorded no change in blood nutrient concentrations, there was no change in frequency of violence. In the sixteen who had beneficial changes in nutrient status, the results were remarkable. They had committed 131 violent acts at baseline, and this went down to eleven during intervention. More recently, Dr. Bernard Gesch from the University of Oxford followed up on the work of Stephen Schoenthaler. In the landmark study, published in the *British Journal of Psychiatry* (2002), his team evaluated the influence of a multivitamin/mineral supplement and essential fatty acids (versus placebos) on the behavior of incarcerated young adults. The active group received the basic multi and four capsules of an omega-6 and omega-3 blend for about five months, while the other half received placebos. There was a total of 231 detainees aged eighteen to twenty-one, most of whom were spending long sentences for serious offenses. Participants taking actual supplements were 26.3 percent less likely to be reported for antisocial behavior versus the placebo group. In those taking supplements, there was a more than 35 percent reduction in offenses compared to the levels at baseline. Despite what appeared to be a balanced offering of dietary choices, a high percentage of detainees consumed (on average) less than the U.K. guidelines for a number of minerals. For example, 97 percent did not consume enough selenium, 74 percent were short on magnesium and potassium, 73 percent were under the iodine recommendations, and 66 percent were low on zinc. Individually, in deficiency, all of these nutrients can disturb mood and behavior. The combined deficiency (even marginal) appeared to have significant consequences in aggression and inappropriate behavior.

What about healthy young adults who are not violent detainees; can multivitamins make a difference? This question has also been addressed in a number of studies, and regular use does appear to make a difference in mood and mental acuity among average folks. In the journal *Psychopharmacology* (1995), Dr. Benton and colleagues showed that a daily multivitamin containing ten times the recommended daily dose of nine vitamins could improve cognitive function. The placebo-controlled study lasted for one year, after which it was the female group who improved more significantly while on the vitamin regimen. Dr. Benton published a separate 1995 study in the journal *Neuropsychobiology* which showed that the same vitamin regimen improved mood in otherwise healthy subjects. Improvements in mood and cognition in these studies were related to corrections in low levels of B vitamins.

In 2000, investigators from the University of Birmingham, U.K., looked at the effect of a multivitamin/mineral combination on psychological well-being. Writing in the journal *Psychopharmacology,* Dr. Douglas Carroll and colleagues showed that the vitamin and mineral combination decreased fatigue, perceived stress, and anxiety in healthy adults. In addition, the group taking the supplement had improved cognitive functioning after one month compared to those taking a placebo. In a study published in *Psychology and Health* (1995), researchers looked at the effects of a basic multivitamin/mineral (and 40 mg ginseng) on the quality of life of midlevel managers. The placebo-controlled study involved 180 healthy men and women, all of whom provided details on typical dietary habits. When the researchers broke down the data, it was the employees who were in the "poor diet" category and actual supplement group who responded well. Compared to placebo, these folks had improvements in tension-anxiety, anger hostility, cognitive function, and overall mood. Even those with a good baseline diet who were in the actual supplement group showed improvements in vigor and perceived stress.

Another area of consideration when it comes to multivitamins is the effect on the immune chemicals that promote inflammation. Remember our old friend IL-6? It is the cytokine that can promote inflammation, compromise brain function, and negatively affect mood. IL-6 is intricately involved in the promotion of cardiovascular disease. There is now a host of studies showing that psychological stressors, including those testy daily hassles, can elevate IL-6 levels. A real problem is that IL-6 levels take a few hours to drop down after an acute stressor, so the saber-toothed tiger causes damage even hours after he disappears. Even worse is that we appear not to extinguish IL-6 elevations after acute stressors are repeated. In other words when it comes to IL-6, we don't adapt well to the same types of stressors when they are regularly applied. So the daily traffic and office grind may continuously elevate IL-6 when these situations are perceived as stress.

Dr. Edward Suarez of Duke University found that IL-6 levels are associated with anger, hostility, and severity of depressive symptoms among non-multivitamin users. In those taking a regular multivitamin, IL-6 concentrations were not associated with these psychological risk factors for cardiovascular disease. Among men who do have anger, hostility, and depressive symptoms, the regular use of multivitamins is associated with lower IL-6 levels—suggesting that multivitamins may have far-reaching health benefits among select groups of otherwise healthy adults.

In order to support the multivitamin stance, one can also look to studies on early childhood allergies (atopy) and asthma. Very young children with atopy have an increased risk of developing major depression or ADHD later in life. The risk of each condition is almost threefold in children with atopy. A new study also shows that kindergarten aged children with asthma are at a much higher risk of having anxiety or depressive symptoms as teenagers. Early childhood atopy and asthma may be associated with deficiencies of omega-3 fatty acids, certain vitamins and minerals, and dietary antioxidants. The makeup of the intestinal bacterial flora may also be a common thread—with allergic children having diminished levels of beneficial bacteria. Pediatric recurrent abdominal pain and infantile colic have been found to be associated with behavioral problems later in life. Recurrent abdominal pain in childhood predicts later anxiety and depressive disorders. A recent study showed that in cases of pediatric colic, the levels of beneficial intestinal bacteria are lower than in healthy controls. The point is that physical conditions that may also be nutritionally influenced in fetal development and early childhood can manifest as brain conditions later on. So, an ounce of prevention is worth a pound in cure.

I know I spent a fair bit of time discussing the value of a multivitamin and mineral formula, but connecting the scientific dots is important so that you can see the valuable picture that emerges.

Essential Fatty Acids

We have already discussed the current situation of overconsumption of oils such as soybean, safflower, sunflower, and corn relative to omega-3 containing fats. Given that the brain is 60 percent fat, and given the wealth of research on the value of omega-3 fatty acids in the brain (and

National Academy of Sciences, Institute of Medicine, Recommended Upper Limits of Adult Dietary Reference Intakes			
Folic acid	1000 mcg	Iodine	1100 mcg
Niacin	35 mg	Iron	45 mg
Vitamin B6	100 mg	Magnesium	350 mg
Vitamin A	3,000 mcg	Manganese	11 mg
Vitamin C	2000 mg	Molybdenum	2000 mcg
Vitamin D	50 mcg	Nickel	1 mg
Vitamin E	1000 mg	Phosphorus	4000 mg
Choline	3500 mg	Selenium	400 mcg
Boron	20 mg	Vanadium	1.8 mg
Calcium	2500 mg	Zinc	40 mg
Copper	10 mg	Water	3.7 litres male
Fluoride	10 mg		2.7 L female

beyond), supplementation should be considered. When it comes to supplementing, I prefer fish oil because the brain-friendly EPA and DHA are already present in the oil. When you use flaxseed oil, perilla, or hemp oil, the parent omega-3 (alpha-linolenic acid) must be converted into EPA and DHA. We can convert, but we are not great at it. For example, a study published in the journal *Lipids* (1999) showed that it takes more than 15 g of alpha-linolenic acid to raise the blood platelet EPA levels compared to just 70 mg of preformed EPA per day. Given that flax oil is 50 percent alpha-linolenic acid, and that one tablespoon holds about 14 g of oil, this research suggests that it would take 14 or 15 tablespoons of flax oil to provide the mood-regulating effects of 500 mg of pure EPA from fish oil.

The current combined intake of brain-critical EPA and DHA is around 130 mg. For most North Americans it is not even close to where we need to be. The international panel of lipid experts recommended a minimum of 650 mg. If you are not regularly consuming salmon, sardines, mackerel, and anchovies, supplementation may be advised.

Many pediatricians are now recommending fish oils during pregnancy for optimal brain development. While the research shows that fish oils, and EPA in particular, can help regulate mood later in life, the DHA is critical as building blocks of the brain in fetal development and early life.

Emerging research is also showing that DHA may help maintain that brain structure over the long term and help stave off dementia. Eating fish just once per week reduces the risk of Alzheimer's by 60 percent.

A new animal study published in the *Proceedings of the National Academy of Sciences* (2005) showed that early life omega-3 deficiency can cause abnormal zinc metabolism in the brain later in life. These same zinc abnormalities may be setting Alzheimer's disease in motion. Omega-3 fatty acids and fish oil supplements are very important throughout life; however, the emerging research suggests that pregnancy and early development sets the tone for life. Gamma-linolenic acid (GLA) is an omega-6 fatty acid derived from evening primrose oil, borage oil, and blackcurrant seed oil. It is quite different from the other omega-6 oils such as corn, safflower, sunflower, and soybean, which contain no GLA. In contrast, GLA has the ability to dampen down the inflammatory pathways by reducing PGE2, a well-known inflammatory chemical. GLA has been shown to be of value in a number of medical conditions, most notably arthritis. In new studies showing the value of essential fatty acids in childhood impulsivity disorders, GLA appears to add to the effectiveness of fish oil. GLA has also been successfully combined with fish oil in the treatment of chronic fatigue syndrome.

Probiotics

The term *probiotic therapy* generally refers to the use of viable bacteria to positively influence the health of the gastrointestinal tract. As we reviewed in chapter 6, the value of beneficial bacteria inside the intestines may have far-reaching effects way beyond the gut. In fact, the microbes of the intestinal tract may be influencing neurotransmission and behavior. The research in this area is finally starting to gather momentum, and hopefully further research will determine if the administration of probiotics in yogurt or capsules will benefit brain conditions.

I will go on record as feeling confident that probiotics will prove to be of value in some brain conditions. The reason I feel optimistic is that certain strains of bacteria can dampen inflammation and provide antioxidant protection outside the gut. While researchers sort things out, the large volumes of international research supporting *Lactobacilli* and *Bifidobacteria* in human health, combined with the observations that the intestinal bacteria is altered in some brain-related conditions, are more than enough to consider probiotics as a worthwhile supplement.

A recent study in the *Journal of Clinical Gastroenterology* (2005) highlights the evidence for probiotics in human health. Researchers from Yale University and the University of Connecticut identified 288 outcomes in human clinical trials published between 1980 and August 2004. Incredibly, they found that there were 239 positive outcomes noted, and only 49 negative or no-effect results. The vast majority of the studies used just a single strain of bacteria, while only 60 used multiple bacterial strains. Among the results, 10 outcome measurements examined certain strains of bacteria on lactose intolerance—in 8 of these 10 outcome measurements, probiotics positively influenced lactose intolerance. I find this very, very interesting when you consider the emerging research on lactose intolerance and depression.

Researchers in different European countries have shown that fructose and lactose malabsorption are associated with early signs of depression, and in those actually with depression, the prevalence of lactose and fructose intolerance was 71 percent compared to just 15 percent in healthy controls. Lactose and fructose intolerance have the potential to influence mood and brain function because they lead to lowered folic acid, zinc, and blood tryptophan levels. They also set the stage for small intestinal bacterial overgrowth.

Dietary interventions are of course priority number one, and clinician-supervised lactose and fructose restricted diets have been shown to lead to remarkable improvements. Drs. Stephanie Matthews and

In addition to dairy, here are some examples of hidden lactose sources:

- Cakes, cookies, bread, and other baked products
- Weight loss powders
- Processed breakfast foods and drinks
- Instant foods
- Butter replacement spreads
- Luncheon meats
- Dips and salad dressings
- Soups and sauces

Anthony Campbell from Cardiff, U.K., have reported improvements in a wide range of non-gastrointestinal symptoms when lactose was removed. Based on the research of these doctors, many cases of chronic unexplained illnesses, including those that might fill the criteria for chronic fatigue syndrome, irritable bowel syndrome, depression, and anxiety, may indeed be lactose intolerance. They have a new guidebook (*Tony's Lactose Free Cookbook*) to assist those with lactose intolerance in making healthy choices.

Dr. Maximilian Ledochowski from the University of Innsbruck, Austria, showed that a fructose reduced diet improved depressive symptoms by more than 65 percent in those who had high levels of hydrogen on breath tests. When lactose and fructose reach the colon unabsorbed, they are acted on by bacteria to produce hydrogen. The same thing happens in small intestinal bacterial overgrowth, except in that case, the lactose and fructose never get a chance to be fully absorbed. Interestingly, blood levels of zinc are low in cases of fructose malabsorption, and low zinc levels are associated with depression and the inability to metabolize the parent omega-3 fatty acid into EPA and DHA.

If you have a variety of gastrointestinal complaints along with mood, cognitive or other brain-related symptoms and/or fatigue and muscle ache, I strongly suggest you see a health-care provider to have the lactulose hydrogen breath test performed. It is simple and noninvasive, and while not 100 percent accurate, it can determine if you have bacterial overgrowth and may eliminate the need to have separate lactose and fructose tolerance tests.

In addition to lactose and fructose restricted diets, many experts recommend probiotics to address dietary sugar intolerances and small intestinal bacterial overgrowth. One of the most significant problems with probiotics is finding a brand that has therapeutic levels of viable bacteria inside the bottle, or the yogurt container. There have been a number of reports in the United States and Canada where independent testing has revealed that there are few, if any, live bacteria in commercial pills, powders, and yogurts. In addition, the beneficial effects of probiotics appear to be very much related to the strain of bacteria involved. Sadly, probiotics are still marketed under the umbrella term "acidophilus," and consumers are led to believe that any old probiotic (or acidophilus) will do. That is clearly not the case, and consumers should know that there are three important parts to a probiotic name—genus, species, and strain. For example, two of the more researched strains in the world are *Lactobacillus* (genus) *casei* (species) Shirota (strain) and *Lactobacillus* (genus) *plantarum* (species) 299V (strain). These are well-documented bacterial strains that have been subjected to scientific and medical research. See the Appendix for recommended probiotics.

Fiber

As previously discussed, it is a challenge for most North Americans to consume the recommended amounts of dietary fiber. We are about 33 percent lower on the fiber scale compared to what was consumed in traditional diets just a century ago. Depending on age and gender, North Americans are on the average 7 to 25 grams short of optimal intake. The recommendations on fiber are based on solid research showing a protective effect against heart disease. The cardiovascular arena has been the focus of decades of nutritional research, while only more recently has the diet-brain connection been given adequate attention. An interesting and consistent message has emerged—what is good for the heart is good for the brain. The same inflammatory chemicals and immune cytokines that cause damage to blood vessels also chip away at brain cells.

Dietary fiber has always been considered heart healthy because it has a modest effect on cholesterol. The benefits of fiber appear to go way beyond cholesterol lowering; new research shows that dietary fiber has significant anti-inflammatory properties. Inflammation has been a constant theme in this book; it is clearly involved in the vicious cycle of attack on the brain. Inflammation on neurodegenerative diseases such as Alzheimer's and Parkinson's diseases has been known for years. More recently, researchers have found that chronic, low-level inflammation is also characteristic of depression and anxiety disorders. Many doctors now look at C-reactive protein (CRP), an inflammatory marker, to examine the risk of cardiovascular disease. Research published in the *Archives of Internal Medicine* (2004) showed a strong association between CRP levels and a history of depression in men. Following this, Spanish researchers reported in the *International Journal of Neuropsychopharmacology* (2005) that CRP levels are higher in panic disorder. While researchers sort out whether such associations are cause, effect, or both in depression and anxiety, what you should know is that fiber can lower CRP. In one study, cardiovascular patients were placed on a diet whereby fiber increased from 14 to 32 g per day. CRP levels were decreased by more than 40 percent during the course of two years on the fiber-rich diet. In a study published in the *Journal of Nutrition* (2004), researchers showed that among almost four thousand subjects, those with the lowest dietary fiber intake had a 50 percent higher risk of having elevated levels of CRP versus those with high fiber intake.

Dr. Dana King of the Medical University of South Carolina and colleagues reported similar results in the *American Journal of Cardiology* (2003). In this case, the elevation of CRP was significantly lower (50 percent) among those in the highest fiber group. Dr. King's group is now conducting a large study to determine the effects of fiber supplements on CRP.

An interesting study published in the journal *Nutrition* (2005) made scientists sit up and take notice of the diets of those who attempt suicide. The researchers studied a group of more than four hundred adults who had a lifetime history of suicide attempts. They found that there were only two nutritional differences between them and controls without such history—low polyunsaturated fat intake and low fiber intake. The polyunsaturated connection makes sense because these are omega-3 fatty acids, but what about fiber? Dietary fiber is a marker of more nutritious whole grains, fruits and vegetables, foods that supply brain-critical vitamins, minerals, and antioxidant phytonutrients. Dietary fiber also promotes the growth of beneficial intestinal bacteria, which in turn may have direct and indirect effects on the central nervous system. It is also possible that dietary fiber may lower the inflammatory cascade and prevent immune chemicals from disturbing neurotransmission. Hopefully Dr. King's work on fiber and inflammation will shed further light on this connection. In the meantime, dietary fiber in the form of fruits, vegetables, and whole grains should be maximized, and supplementation should be considered for some adults.

Fiber Caveat?

Now that I have devoted pages of this book extolling the benefits of fiber, you might ask what possible caveats could there be? Well, for starters, individuals with irritable bowel syndrome may want to be cautious about fiber. While fiber is purported to be the "cure" for IBS, there is absolutely no convincing evidence that this is the case. In fact, some studies have shown that fiber reductions, or avoidance of certain types of fiber including bran, might actually improve IBS. The most recent study, published in *Digestive Diseases and Sciences* (2005), showed that a fiber-restricted diet significantly reduced abdominal symptoms. In addition, the fiber-restricted diet cut the hydrogen and methane gas production by more than half. Dr. Keith Dear and colleagues conclude, "The perception by some IBS patients that their symptoms are due to excessive gas may be correct. Treatments aimed at reducing fermentation, such as a low-fiber diet, may alleviate symptoms in many patients."

There is also another concern regarding excessive fermentation in the large intestine, and that is production of lactic acids. Lactate was first discovered and isolated from sour milk in 1780, and it comes in two near-identical forms, D-lactate and L-lactate. The L-lactate is found in the blood of humans because it is produced by our cells in metabolic processes. The D-lactate is present only at minuscule (nanomolar) concentrations in healthy adults. D-lactate is produced inside the colon when remaining carbohydrates are delivered from the small intestine. D-lactate levels are kept low by the activities of intestinal bacteria, which convert D-lactate into acetate. Normal gastric emptying, optimal small intestinal digestion and absorption of carbohydrates, and normal intestinal microflora are all prerequisites to keeping everything in balance. If there is poor digestion of carbohydrates in the small intestine, or if for any reason sugars and fermentable carbohydrates are being dumped into the colon in excessive fashion, lactic acid can reveal its nasty side. The consequences of delivering excess sugars to the colon have been well documented in patients who have had portions of their small intestines surgically removed or bypassed. The colon becomes acidic, acid-resistant bacteria overgrow, and lactic acid production is stepped up more than a few notches.

When D-lactate production exceeds our ability to clear it, a host of neurological and psychiatric symptoms are the result. While gastroenterologists were writing up their findings about D-lactate-induced changes in their patients, researchers in the psychiatric arena were consistently reporting that I.V. lactate can induce anxiety and panic attacks.

In 2000, a study in *Biological Psychiatry* showed that I.V. lactate elicited intense emotional responses in perpetrators of domestic violence. These individuals (both males and females) showed more lactate-induced rage and panic, and showed greater changes in speech, breathing, and motor activity than did nonviolent control subjects. While there have been some theories put forward, there is no widely accepted mechanism to explain why lactic acids disturbs cognition and behavior. Could it be that a carbohydrate overload in the colon could induce panic and behavioral disturbances in individuals who have never had intestinal surgery? What about those with intestinal motility problems, what about the research on fructose and lactose malabsorption lowering typtophan and setting the table for psychiatric disorder? Is it really far-fetched to wonder if, in some folks, unabsorbed sugar, fermentable carbohydrates, and altered microflora might be combining to chronically produce more lactate than they can handle?

As a brain-oriented nutritional scientist, and as a clinician observing the effects of fiber on certain individuals, I have been asking these questions for a number of years. Apparently, I wasn't the only one. Dr. Edward Clayton and colleagues from Sydney, Australia, performed an elegant study showing that fiber-induced fermentation in the colons of rats was associated with increased anxiety and aggression. Writing in the journal *Physiology and Behavior* (2004), these researchers showed that intestinal lactic acid, both L-lactate and D-lactate, as well as another potentially brain-toxic fermentation product called propionate, were all involved in the behavioral disturbances. This study is a massive call to further investigate intestinal lactic acid production in those with brain conditions. In the meantime, if you feel that you are sensitive to dietary fiber, there are commercially available noninvasive tests to examine D-lactate breakdown in urine. See the Appendix for more details.

Antioxidants

A substantial amount of space in these pages has been devoted to highlighting the consistent finding that brain conditions are associated with oxidative stress. It would then seem reasonable that taking an isolated antioxidant pill would be a wise move. The only problem with that line of thinking is that isolated antioxidants have yielded mixed findings when it comes to brain health. Individual antioxidants, such as vitamin C and E, are pretty weak when it comes to clinical research, or even downright dangerous according to some research on vitamin E and beta-carotene. Taken in high doses alone, isolated antioxidants have the potential to act as pro-oxidants. They are called *biphasic*, meaning that at a certain level they actually contribute to oxidative stress when they are not supported by other members of the antioxidant family. Yes, they actually worsen the situation.

As mentioned previously, antioxidants work together, much like an orchestra, and one antioxidant can negate the pro-oxidant effects of another. Research also shows that two antioxidants together have greater antioxidant potential than the sum of the two individually. Not only are vitamin-based antioxidant supplements like vitamin E and beta-carotene potentially harmful, they really don't seem to work well when used alone as supplements. You see greater effects when supplements are combined. My attitude is similar when it comes to botanical remedies. Research on gingko, ginseng, bilberry, grape extracts, and other botanicals is encouraging, but are you really going to take all these supplements for the rest of your life? Would you even want to?

The availability of whole fruit, vegetable, and herbal extracts as powder is an exciting development in the supplement world. Modern extraction techniques can remove the water from fruits, vegetables, and herbs while leaving the nutrients behind. The powdered supplements in this category are generally referred to as "green food" supplements. They have been popular in Japan for decades. The first successful green food product introduced into North America was that by nutrition researcher Sam Graci. The product in question, greens+, was the subject of two impressive clinical studies.

The first study, published in the *Canadian Journal of Dietetic Practice and Research* (2004), involved more than one hundred otherwise healthy women from Toronto. They were instructed to take either greens+ or a carefully matched (placebo) powdered beverage for three months. Subjects were evaluated using various validated questionnaires. Those taking the actual greens+ were found to have improvements in vitality and significantly more energy than those in the placebo group. These are very encouraging results.

In separate research, University of Toronto researchers found that greens+ increased blood antioxidant levels and lowered oxidative stress in otherwise healthy adults. According to Dr. Venket Rao and his team, the beneficial phytonutrients (polyphenols) in greens+ are well absorbed. This is an important finding because research has shown that polyphenols are not always well absorbed. Finally, new University of Toronto research has shown that greens+ stimulates osteoblasts, the cells which are critical in bone formation and maintenance. This is also an important consideration given the emerging research on bone mineral loss in brain conditions, including Alzheimer's disease and depression. I'm not suggesting for one minute that greens+ or any other green food supplement is a substitute for a plate full of colorful fruits and vegetables. It is, however, a good insurance policy to ensure adequate intake of a variety of health-promoting phytochemicals.

Many of the ingredients in greens+, and similar products in the category, have a reputation for being brain protective. A product such as greens+ allows consistent intake of low to moderate levels of herbs over an extended period of time in an effort to take advantage of a synergistic effect. These green food products avoid megadoses of any particular ingredient; instead they supply a blend of much needed phytochemicals and nutrients that are obviously absent from the average North American diet.

What's in greens+?

Phosphatide complex (phosphatidyl choline from lecithin)

Organic alfalfa, barley, wheat grass & red beet powder

Spirulina

Apple pectin

Japanese chlorella

Organic soy sprouts

Organic whole brown rice powder

Stevia leaf powder

Non-dairy bacterial cultures containing *Lactobacilli* and *Bifidobacteria*

Royal jelly

Bee pollen

Full spectrum grape extract

Licorice root extract

Acerola berry juice powder

Siberian ginseng extract

Milk thistle extract

Organic Nova Scotia dulse powder

Ginkgo biloba extract

Japanese green tea extract

European bilberry extract

Other Supplements

The basics of supplementation for brain health include the consideration of a multivitamin/mineral, essential fatty acids, probiotics, fiber, and a green food supplement. The following are some other supplements that have gained popularity as brain-boosting, and stress-busting nutrients and herbs. Remember that there is no fountain of youth in a bottle, be it a supplement bottle or a wine bottle. I saw the headlines too: "Life extending chemical found in red wine," *New York Times* (August 24, 2003), and others like it. The Japanese are the longest lived people on earth, and they are not the largest consumers of a red wine that is made in cool climates, nor are they popping resveratrol in large quantities—the isolated phytochemical thought to be the longevity factor. These sensational headlines are based on extending the life span of yeast and fruit flies; humans are much more complex and require a multi-nutrient intervention for longevity. Again, taking a green food supplement with whole red grape extract, some ginkgo, and other antioxidant botanicals makes more sense from the synergy perspective. Nevertheless, some supplements are worth highlighting and may indeed be worth trying. Condition-specific recommendations will be made later on.

GINKGO BILOBA

The ginkgo tree is known as the living fossil because its history spans some 200 million years on this planet. Ginkgo leaf extract is widely used in Europe for the treatment of various conditions, most notably Alzheimer's disease and dementia. In the mid- to late-1990s, ginkgo caught on rapidly as the memory pill of choice. The thinking was, hey, if ginkgo can improve the memory of those with dementia, just think what it can do for a healthy person. Ginkgo remains one of the best-selling herbs in North America.

As of 2005, close to fifty trials have investigated ginkgo and human cognition. Based on the overall results when the data are pooled, ginkgo does emerge as useful in improving the symptoms of dementia and in treating mild to moderate cognitive deficits in Alzheimer's disease. While results are conflicting, a number of studies have shown that ginkgo can improve memory, mood, alertness, well-being, and quality of life in healthy volunteers. When it comes to memory, the combination of ginseng and ginkgo appears to be a good option according to some published studies. This illustrates my view on synergy of foods and herbs.

Ginkgo biloba appears to work by a number of mechanisms. It is a potent antioxidant, can increase blood flow to the brain, protects nerve cell membranes, and inhibits the buildup of beta-amyloid plaque involved in Alzheimer's disease. Two often overlooked areas of research are ginkgo's influence on essential fatty acids and its influence on cortisol. In 2000, French researchers showed that a commercially available ginkgo extract (EG6 761) could increase the omega-3 (EPA) levels in the membranes of red blood cells. The ginkgo also prevented oxidative damage to red blood cells. In 2002, researchers from Slovakia showed that the same EGB 761 extract could prevent rises in cortisol levels after experimental mental stress.

Gingko is probably most effective as a preventative plant. The evidence related to improvements in dementia are apparent, but they are not huge. If you choose to supplement with ginkgo, I would recommend taking the EGB 761 (sold as Ginkgold) because the vast majority of clinical work has been performed with this extract.

While ginkgo has enjoyed an impressive track record of safety in Europe and North America, it can cause blood thinning at higher doses or if combined with other herbal remedies or drugs. Due to its blood thinning effect, gingko should be discontinued prior to surgery.

ACETYL-L-CARNITINE AND ALPHA-LIPOIC ACID

Although these agents have their own unique properties, the emerging research from Dr. Bruce Ames and colleagues from the University of California suggest that the combination exerts quite an effect. Acetyl-L-carnitine (ALC) is a natural compound found in small amounts in dairy and meat. ALC plays an important role in the energy packet inside our cells, a little fuel-manufacturing facility known as the mitochondria. When mitochondrial function becomes subpar, not only do we feel less energetic, the oxidative stress that results from mitochondrial disturbances serves to play a role in neurological and psychiatric conditions. It is a complicated biochemical story, but ultimately the combination of energy dysregulation and oxidative stress have assumed the spotlight in numerous brain conditions. The gasoline of our cells is called ATP, and ALC helps to prevent the loss of ATP in brain-related conditions. ATP depletion is caused by mitochondrial disturbances, which in turn are caused by oxidative stress, nutritional deficiencies, microbial infections, and a host of other assaults. Mitochondrial abnormalities are known to be a part of chronic fatigue syndrome and the amyloid buildup of Alzheimer's can directly deplete ATP. Individuals with chronic fatigue syndrome have low levels of ALC, and the lower the levels, the more pronounced the fatigue. In chronic fatigue patients, there is also a decreased uptake of ALC in certain regions of the brain. This in turn may influence the manufacture of important mood and behavior regulating neurotransmitters. Animal studies show that ALC can reduce impulsive behavior in a validated model of ADHD. ALC has also been shown to protect animals against the effects of stress, improve memory, and protect nerve cells against damage. In controlled studies, ALC has been reported to have beneficial effects in both major depression and Alzheimer's disease.

Alpha-lipoic acid (ALA) is one of our most potent antioxidants. We discussed it previously with regard to its reported ability to improve mold toxicity. It is known as the universal antioxidant because it works in both water-soluble and fat-soluble environments. Much like acetyl-L-carnitine, ALA works as a co-factor in mitochondrial metabolic reactions that produce energy. As previously mentioned, ALA helps preserve and recycle our other antioxidants, including vitamin C and E, glutathione, and coenzyme Q10. ALA improves blood sugar control and may help to prevent the effects of heavy metal toxicities. Experimentally, ALA has been shown to prevent obesity by regulating an enzyme in the food control center of the brain. The enzyme AMPK is found in the hypothalamus, and when stimulated it promotes food intake. ALA has been shown to keep AMPK in check and aid in weight loss in rodents. Many of the effects of ALA are mediated not by its role as an antioxidant, but rather by other enzymatic mechanisms. In a recent study in the *Journal of Neuroimmunology* (2004), researchers showed that ALA protects against experimental multiple sclerosis. ALA prevented disease progression, significantly reduced damage to the myelin (the outer coat on the nerve cell, which is damaged in MS), and dampened inflammation. These encouraging findings are a call for a clinical trial using ALA in multiple sclerosis.

For more than a decade, Dr. Bruce Ames and his colleagues have been examining ways and means to stop mitochondrial "decay," or at least slow it down. He and his team from the University of California, Berkeley, have consistently found ALC and ALA to be superstars in their ability to keep the mitochondria working in top gear. In fact, they have repeatedly found that ALC and ALA can restore mitochondrial function, lower oxidative stress, and improve mobility and cognition in elderly rats. The researchers have put together an ALC/ALA combination in supplement form, the new product is called Juvenon. I feel compelled to point out that that these researchers are not corporate fat cats trying to cash in on an anti-aging gimmick. They created the supplement out of solid science and have agreed to use the proceeds from sales to fund a controlled clinical trial. Juvenon may be of real value in chronic fatigue syndrome where ALA is low, and oxidative stress is a hallmark of the illness. While we await the results of clinical trials, all arrows point to the combination of ALC and ALA being of benefit in the preservation of brain function and the treatment of brain-related conditions. Both ALC and ALA are generally well tolerated, and there are no known contraindications. Because ALA can help regulate blood sugar, diabetics on medication should report ALA use to physicians.

COENZYME-Q10

Also called ubiquinone, this fat-soluble compound is also involved in the production of the gasoline of human cells—ATP. Much like ALC and ALA, Co-enzyme Q10 is a powerful antioxidant and is particularly effective in protecting the mitochondria. Experimental studies suggest that CoQ10 may be of benefit in protection against cardiovascular disease and, again, given the heart-brain connection, it is no surprise that studies show brain-protective properties too. New clinical studies suggest that CoQ10 is valuable in reducing the symptoms of Parkinson's disease and reducing the frequency of migraine headaches.

5-HYDROXYTRYPTOPHAN AND SEROTONIN-BOOSTERS

Serotonin, the so-called "feel-good" brain chemical, is manufactured from the amino acid L-tryptophan. Antidepressant drugs work by keeping more serotonin around for use at the nerve cells—they usually work by preventing the breakdown of serotonin and/or preventing it from being placed back in storage. A limited number of studies have shown that L-tryptophan may be helpful in treating depressive symptoms, anxiety, and insomnia and that it generally promotes a calming effect or mild sedation. However, a contaminated batch of L-tryptophan from Japan was likely responsible for serious illness in more than 1,500 people and an estimated 30 deaths. The illness, eosinophilia myalgia syndrome (EMS), resulted in an FDA-issued recall in 1989 and L-tryptophan disappeared from the North American over-the-counter market.

Another related supplement (one step closer to serotonin) became a suitable replacement—5-hydroxytryptophan or 5-HTP for short. L-tryptophan gets converted into 5-HTP, which in turn gets converted into serotonin. 5-HTP has the advantage of readily passing through the highly regulated blood-brain barrier (BBB). Once through the BBB, 5-HTP is taken up by the nerve cells and completely converted into serotonin. As a result, the clinically effective doses of 5-HTP are much lower than those of L-tryptophan (around 200 mg versus 2 to 6 g of L-tryptophan).

There have been a number of clinical trials showing the benefits of 5-HTP in brain-related conditions including panic disorder, depression, insomnia, migraines, and fibromyalgia. Most of these were small clinical trials and the doses of 300 to 400 mg daily would be an expensive way to get results. Despite the benefits, some words of caution regarding 5-HTP are in order. Unless supervised by a doctor, it should not be taken with antidepressants because "serotonin syndrome" or overload of serotonin may result. The symptoms of serotonin syndrome are euphoria, drowsiness, sustained rapid eye movement, overreaction of the reflexes, rapid muscle contraction and relaxation in the ankle causing abnormal movements of the foot, clumsiness, restlessness, feeling drunk and dizzy, muscle contraction and relaxation in the jaw, sweating, intoxication, muscle twitching, rigidity, and high body temperature.

The typical side effects of 5-HTP taken within standard dosages are generally minimal and most often involve digestive upset.

Instead of supplementing with 5-HTP, patients with brain-related conditions may want to consider ingesting natural food-based tryptophan in the form of ZenBev™. This multi-patented product includes pumpkin-seed flour mixed with carbohydrate in the precise ratio required to get the tryptophan up into the brain for conversion to serotonin. Although naturally high in tryptophan, pumpkin seeds alone will generally not be effective in boosting brain serotonin levels. Tryptophan will remain in the blood and not gain access through the blood-brain barrier and into the brain unless a specific ratio of carbohydrate is also consumed.

After years of research, Toronto psychiatrist Dr. Craig Hudson and his team determined that a blend of pumpkinseed flour and carbohydrate can increase serotonin and melatonin for sleep. Early clinical trials using ZenBev™ have shown favorable results in the areas of decreased anxiety and improved sleep. The powdered product, which mixes into a drink, may be a much more effective and practical means to improve the symptoms of certain brain-related symptoms than many 5-HTP capsules. See the Appendix for availability.

Another option to promote sleep and lower stress from a food-based supplement is that of alpha-lactalbumin (ALA), a milk protein. ALA is particularly rich in tryptophan, and new research in the *American Journal of Clinical Nutrition* (2005) showed that ALA taken in the evening led to improved morning alertness and cognitive function the following day. The researchers suggested the effects were due to improved sleep via higher brain serotonin. These results support earlier animal studies showing a sleep-inducing effect of ALA, and human research showing a stress-buffering effect.

RHODIOLA ROSEA

Rhodiola is a new and exciting herb that has only recently come to the North American market. The use of Rhodiola is backed up by solid human studies. Rhodiola has been studied intensively in Russian scientific laboratories over the last forty years. It has been used traditionally to enhance work performance and energy and decrease irritability under stressful conditions, physical and mental strain, and viral exposure. Rhodiola is a classic adaptogen, i.e. a botanical or nutrient that helps an individual adapt to stress.

Two double-blind, placebo-controlled trials of Rhodiola extract appeared in Western scientific journals in 2000. The first study showed that the Rhodiola group (170 mg/day) had statistically significant improvements in mental performance and measures of fatigue versus placebo among medical doctors working night-call rotations. The second trial involved medical students during a stressful exam period. The study showed that those who received 100 mg of Rhodiola had significant improvements in physical fitness, mental performance, sleep patterns, motivation to study, and general well-being. Those taking Rhodiola also reported less need for sleep, greater mood stability, and reductions in mental fatigue versus those on placebo.

In 2003, a joint Russian-Swedish study showed that just one dose of Rhodiola given during stressful conditions could improve mental function versus placebo. This study, again double-blind and placebo-controlled, showed that single doses of Rhodiola given at 4:00 in the morning could improve capacity for mental work and prevented fatigue onset. Also in 2003, researchers showed that Rhodiola helps to maintain the content of ATP in skeletal muscles. ATP is the fuel of all our cells. In addition, Rhodiola keeps blood levels of C-reactive protein in check after exhaustive exercise. Given that C-reactive protein is our most important marker of inflammation, it appears that Rhodiola has a potent anti-inflammatory effect.

There have been no significant side effects noted for Rhodiola at the doses used in the clinical trials. Supplementation with Rhodiola has not been evaluated in pregnancy and lactation and should therefore be avoided during these times.

ST. JOHN'S WORT

This well-known herbal antidepressant has received a significant amount of both positive and negative press over the last few years. Some trials support the botanical and some don't. However, according to a recent review published in the *American Family Physician* (2005), the preponderance of evidence indicates that SJW is effective for mild to moderate depression. Although the efficacy of SJW is similar to that of most antidepressants for non-severe depression, it is associated with far fewer side effects. SJW is generally well tolerated, with 2.4 percent of users reporting an adverse reaction. The most common adverse reactions include gastrointestinal discomfort, insomnia, and headaches. Although it's not commonly reported, skin may also become hypersensitive to sun exposure after administration of SJW.

An area of real concern regarding SJW is when it is co-administered with other drugs. SJW can speed up the elimination of medications from the body due to its effects on drug-metabolizing enzymes in the liver. There are a host of drugs that may be affected by SJW, actually about half of all marketed drugs, including blood-thinning medications and the birth control pill. SJW

• • • **CASE REPORT** • • •

Sandy is a fifty-year-old woman with chronic fatigue syndrome (CFS). Although the formal diagnosis was made only two years ago, the symptoms of post-exertion fatigue, sleep disturbances, headaches, muscle ache, and mental "fog" came on after a winter viral infection seven years earlier. She suffered depression and irritability, mostly as a result of frustration in adapting to this life-altering illness—particularly because Sandy was a very high-functioning individual prior to the onset of CFS.

A diet diary revealed a high-calorie but nutritionally poor diet. There were lots of empty calories, simple carbohydrates, sweets, TV dinners, and "instant" foods loaded with sugars and food additives. Due to the fatigue of the illness, CFS patients often fall into the trap of relying on a quick supply of calories. But inadequate intakes of nutrients and too many chemical additives are tied in with the symptoms of CFS. While food intolerances may be a part of CFS, Sandy had tried removing wheat and dairy with no change in symptoms. She was not a fish eater and ate deli meats on most days. Unlike most CFS patients, she was not taking any supplements, having tried a variety of "immune" herbs without success.

High-antioxidant foods are particularly important for CFS patients, so Sandy was placed on a diet including prepared greens, whole-grain cereals, nuts, yogurt, frozen and canned vegetables for easy preparation, Yakult™ probiotic drink, and dark pigmented fruits including blueberries, acai, and cherries. Processed meats were eliminated; red meat intake was cut back dramatically and replaced with lean poultry and high-omega-3 eggs. Instant foods and prepared foods containing MSG and aspartame were eliminated. A special hypoallergenic whey-based formula (nutrilean+™) that meets government meal replacement criteria was used, not for weight loss, but rather as a convenient small meal.

Supplements were kept to the basics—omega-3 fatty acids in the form of EPA are essential. Sandy was placed on 1000 mg of EPA (o3mega+ joy™) and a daily multivitamin/mineral formula. In addition, to support the possible deficits in cellular energy production in CFS, Sandy began taking 100 mg of co-enzyme Q10 and two capsules of Juvenon™, an acetyl-L-carnitine and alpha-lipoic acid combination. In addition to the supplements, mind-body medicine is a critical component of reducing symptoms in any medical condition where stress can exacerbate the illness. Purposeful physical activity balanced with an awareness of energy conservation is also central to recovery. Sandy did well on her plan, and reported a 60 percent improvement in symptoms after three months. Given the notoriously difficult nature of CFS, this is a substantial gain.

should also not be co-administered with traditional antidepressant medications due to the risk of serotonin syndrome (too much serotonin).

The bottom line with SJW is that it may be effective in improving mild to moderate depression and it has the added value of strong antioxidant activity. The antiviral activity of SJW gets promoted on various Web sites but human studies show no antiviral effect. The EPA concentrate from fish oil (1000 mg) may enhance the effects of SJW. The brand of choice is Perika™ by Nature's Way because it contains the SJW extract used in clinical studies. The dose is typically 300 mg three times a day; however, make sure you discuss SJW and the EPA with your doctor.

S-ADENOSYL METHIONINE

S-adenosyl methionine (SAMe) is arguably the supplement with the highest level of evidence to support its use in the treatment of depressive symptoms and pain-reduction. A number of controlled trials have shown that both oral and intravenous SAMe is of value in the treatment of depression and fibromyalgia. SAMe may also promote restful sleep. SAMe has been shown to support liver detoxification and improve antioxidant status by its ability to increase glutathione levels. Animal research has shown that SAMe can increase serotonin levels throughout the brain and may keep the nerve cells more "fluid" or flexible for proper neurotransmission.

SAMe may be a worthwhile supplement for patients with brain-related conditions—side effects are rare and usually consist of gastrointestinal disturbances, dry mouth, and restlessness. SAMe may have a mild blood-thinning effect. Patients who are taking antidepressant medications or natural products such as 5-hydroxytryptophan, ZenBev™, or Hypericum (St. John's wort) should only take SAMe under direct supervision of a health-care provider. There is one massive practical drawback of SAMe, despite its potential benefits: the therapeutic doses of SAMe are not cheap; when taking the research-based doses of 600 to 800 mg daily, you can anticipate a bill of about $80 to $100 (US) a month.

MELATONIN

Just like the moon and the oceans, our human body is in constant rhythm. These natural circadian rhythms involve waxing and waning of core body temperature and spontaneous muscle (motor) activity.

Melatonin is a hormone secreted by the brain's pineal gland in a twenty-four-hour circadian rhythm, regulating the sleep-wake cycle. Melatonin secretion normally increases about two hours before bedtime, peaks in the middle of the night, and drops thereafter. The rise and fall of melatonin is critical to the quality of human sleep. Research has shown that melatonin administration can enhance sleep when taken six hours before the natural peak. So that would be 10:00 p.m., assuming a natural peak of 4:00 a.m.

Note that melatonin taken in the morning can cause dizziness, drowsiness, and diminished daytime alertness. The research has focused mostly on insomnia due to shift work or jet lag. Interestingly, recent research has shown that melatonin is a potent antioxidant and has synergistic activity when co-administered with vitamins C and E. Experimental studies show that melatonin can prevent the negative effects of oxidative stress induced by cellular phones. New research shows that melatonin may be helpful in fibromyalgia and in reducing the pain of irritable bowel syndrome.

Remember that hormones work much like an orchestra: individual hormones can have a tremendous effect on the manufacture and secretion of other hormones. If you are considering giving melatonin a try, please see your health-care provider.

TAURINE

Taurine is a sulfur-containing amino acid essential for the normal electrical working of the brain. It has been shown to be a potent antioxidant within the brain and nervous system. Specifically, taurine helps to prevent damage to the lipid (fat) components of the nerve cells. A number of animal studies show that taurine helps prevent the free-radical damage normally induced by a diet high in sugar. It also increases exercise time, probably because it slows down the buildup of lactic acid within the muscles. Taurine levels have been noted to be low in both Alzheimer's and Parkinson's patients.

Human research shows that taurine supplementation (versus placebo) can cut down on fatigue related to computer work. Taurine helped to lower visual stress and eye strain after extended time spent working in front of a computer monitor. At least four studies have shown that the combination of 1000 mg taurine and 80 mg caffeine (about one cup of coffee) can significantly improve endurance, mental focus, and memory and decrease fatigue in otherwise healthy adults. This combination of taurine and caffeine is the basis of most North American commercial energy drinks. Keep in mind that even small cans of energy drinks come with close to 30 grams of sugar or a solid dose of aspartame—not the ideal delivery format for brain health.

GINSENG

Ginseng, in its three main varieties, American, Asian, and Siberian, remains among the most popular of all herbal remedies. Ginseng is known as the great adaptogen, meaning that it can help humans adapt to, and recover from, acute and chronic stress. There are many experimental animal studies indicating that ginseng enhances energy. In humans, five clinical trials have shown that ginseng improves mood, reaction time, attention, and information processing. The most recent study, published in the *Journal of Psychopharmacology* (2005), showed that ginseng improves performance and staves off feelings of mental fatigue during sustained mental activity.

Although ginseng is marketed primarily for enhanced physical performance and endurance, these claims are not backed up by human research. Despite what you may see on the Internet and in some books, there is no research showing that after one to two months of use, SG needs to be discontinued for two weeks in order to be efffective. When taken at high levels as a solo supplement, ginseng may have caffeine-like side effects, which include anxiety and insomnia.

Summary

We have covered a lot of ground here, yet the supplements we have discussed are just a few among twenty-nine thousand. Obviously, many if not most of these supplements are of little value to the health of the human brain. Many are promoted like they are the magic potion that cures everything and transforms the lives of all who use the product. It is absurd. Individuals with brain disorders, neurological or psychiatric, are desperate and vulnerable to the supplement sharks. It is sad that the bogus claims and unscrupulous marketing of some products obscure the science behind the supplements that really *can* make a huge difference in the life of those seeking optimal brain functioning. Anecdotal evidence and testimonials of cures of brain conditions with an extract from the bark of a tree, or what have you, do nothing to promote common supplement sense. I know I am a little touchy about the overselling of supplements, but as a naturopathic doctor trying to promote the science of supplements, I find that some in mainstream medicine look at me as if I was the one telling the world that coral calcium is the only way to get your calcium. I have also consulted with many patients with chronic illness, the majority of which would (and sometimes do) spend their life savings on the new supplement that is going to be "the one."

When it comes to supplements there are three general rules to follow: They are never a substitute for a colorful and varied diet. They are never a substitute for appropriate medical care. Choose supplements to cover all the basics of nutrition.

The basic supplements are a multivitamin/mineral formula, essential fatty acids, probiotics, fiber (in most cases), and a green (phytonutrient) food formula. Once these basics are squared away, experimentation with dietary supplements for brain-specific conditions or general maintenance may be a worthwhile venture.

9

The Changing Japanese Diet and the Importance of Breakfast

In this chapter, we will introduce some easy brain-friendly recipes. Hopefully this will give you an idea of how easy and delicious it can be fuel and protect your brain. Of course my nutrition consultant from Tokyo, Yoshiko Sato, who developed the meals, has given us a Japanese flavor—and why not? The Japanese are not only the longest-lived people on the planet, they are also much less likely to have many of the brain conditions (neurological and psychiatric) that are common in the West. Dramatic changes to the traditional Japanese diet are rapidly occurring, and the rates of brain-related conditions there are also on the rise. Overall, however, the Japanese diet is still far superior to the North American diet. The graphs peppered throughout this book show that when it comes to a high consumption of sugars, meat, animal fats, vegetable oils, and white potato, North Americans are still leaps and bounds ahead of the Japanese.

Sadly though, the gap is being narrowed, and as American fast-food chains pop up in Japan like dandelions on a lawn, young people are being lured in with the inexpensive taste of animal fat and sugar. Competitive pricing has kept the cost of fast food way down in Japan, and the dietary changes may be taking their toll. The rapidly changing Japanese diet represents one of the largest nutritional experiments in human history, and so far it seems the Westernization of the Japanese diet has not been a good thing.

The Japanese are clearly concerned about the behavioral changes within its society. Sensational headlines have appeared in recent years, such as "School kids becoming more violent" (*Japan Times*, August 28, 2004), "Hokkaido kids hit by depression" (*Japan Times* November 2, 2004), "Tokyo public health experts concerned about 'hikikomori'" (*Lancet* March 30, 2002), and "Poll finds growing crime concern" (*Japan Times* September 19, 2004). Hikikomori is the rapidly growing trend of Japanese youth to completely withdraw from society. Reports suggest that up to one million young Japanese are shutting themselves in their rooms, primarily to avoid stressful situations. Children in the once well-controlled schools are becoming increasingly violent. The Japanese Education ministry has been collecting statistics on violence in public schools since 1997. Since then there has been a consistent increase in violence. In 2003, there was a 5 percent increase in violent acts within the entire school system, and an incredible 28 percent increase in violent acts among elementary school kids.

In the largest study of Japanese children to date, it was shown that almost a quarter of junior high school students suffer from depression as defined by international standards, and one in five exhibits possible suicidal symptoms. Almost 8 percent of elementary school kids showed strong emotional links to depression. These numbers are much higher than rates previously described in children and adults.

The behavior of adults is changing, too; the suicide rate in Japan has doubled since the 1970s and early 1980s. Every year since 1998, more than thirty thousand Japanese have been driven to suicide. A similar pattern has emerged with regard to crime, especially violent crime, in Japan. The crime rate held steady for years in Japan from the 1950s through the 1980s. In the last ten years, however, there has been an incredible 150 percent increase in crime inside Japan. Sadly, Japan is rapidly losing its reputation as the safest developed nation in the world.

What is happening? How could behavior sour so quickly in Japan? There are countless theories: economic recession, the malaise and lethargy of a hyper-commercial society, changing social patterns, foreign influences, antiquated police structure, and others. Since no one seems to be pointing a finger at nutritional influences, let me do so here. I'm not suggesting, even for a minute, that Western dietary influences have alone produced Japan's current situation. Clearly there are multiple factors involved. However, given the nutritional influences on brain and behavior we have discussed in this book so far, from vitamins and minerals to fish oil, is it really that far-fetched to imagine that the rapidly changing Japanese diet might be a contributing factor in influencing behavior? I think not. As French culinary expert Jean Brillat-Savarin stated almost two centuries ago in his famous book, *The Physiology of Taste* (1825), "The destiny of nations depends on the manner in which they nourish themselves." Based on what is happening in Japan and elsewhere, his words ring true today.

In an eye-opening article published almost thirty years ago in the journal *Preventive Medicine* (1978), Dr. Yasuo Kagawa introduced to westerners the incredible longevity of the Japanese living in Okinawa. They had the lowest total caloric, sugar, and salt intakes. Among Japanese, already known for general longevity, Okinawans had the highest rate of individuals who were more than one hundred years old. Dr. Kagawa also showed that the Western diet was bringing with it significant increases in breast, colon, and lung cancers. In 1978 when Dr. Kagawa penned his landmark paper, Japan was only on the cusp of a fast-food explosion. The first American fast-food franchise in Japan had only appeared just two years before in 1976. Ironically, that first American franchised fast-food establishment in Japan wasn't in Tokyo, it was opened in Okinawa, the world's epicenter of longevity.

As incomes grew in the 1980s and '90s, so too did the waistlines of the Okinawans. In fact, as reported in the *New York Times* article "On U.S. Fast Food, More Okinawans Grow Super-Sized" (March 30, 2004), Okinawans are now the heaviest of all Japanese and spend a considerable portion of their income on fast and processed food. No longer are Okinawan men at the top of the longevity list within Japan, they are now actually in the bottom half of the rankings within all of Japan's prefectures.

The older Okinawans still hold on to the traditional diet, low in animal fat, sugar, and preservatives and high in fruits and vegetables. The young do not. The writing was on the wall, or should I say in the pages of *Preventative Medicine*, almost thirty years ago. However, even Dr. Kagawa couldn't have imagined that the Western fast-food industry, just budding in 1976, would grow to such colossal proportions. Maybe he didn't read the words of McDonald's founder Ray Kroc five years earlier in *Time* magazine (September 17, 1973), commenting on his then $500 million fortune: "I expect money like you walk into a room and turn on a light switch or a faucet, it's not enough." In 2003, the Japanese fast-food market was 14.8 billion (U.S.) dollars.

During the economic struggles of the late 1990s, and early 2000s, the Japanese did not turn away from fast food, they ate it up. As reported by Shane Stiles in "Fast Food Feeds Japan's Deflation" (*Gate 39 Media*, 2002), the prices of fast foods were slashed in Japan during this time. This drove up demand. From 1996 to 2001, the price of the leading American fast-food burger sold in Japan actually fell by 18 percent. In 2001, the sales of Japan's leading hamburger, the McDonald's hamburger, went from 250,000 hamburgers per day to 1.25 million burgers per day due to a work-week price slash. I'm not pointing a finger at McDonald's—too many people have already done that, and they are not the cause of our dietary habits. There are countless homegrown Japanese fast-food joints

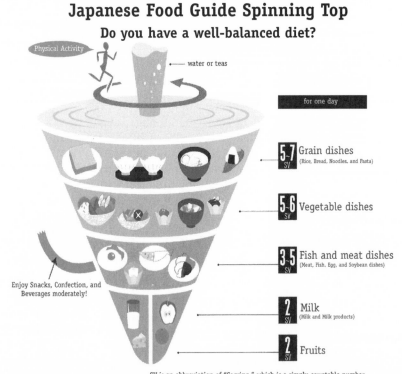

Japanese Food Guide Spinning Top, 2005. Courtesy of the Japanese Ministry of Health, Labour, and Welfare.

now serving up high-calorie, brain un-friendly foods, and no one is making a movie about them. The reality is that prices on all fast food—from sandwiches to pizza to fried chicken—dropped, driving up demand in a recessed Japanese economy.

The Westernization of the Japanese diet is now happening at a lightning pace. New studies are showing that the blood cholesterol of Americans and Japanese is now only marginally different. The last few decades have seen an eightfold increase in saturated fat consumption, and red meat intake has more than tripled over the last thirty years. The increase in processed food consumption has increased by well over 200 percent since 1970.

In a thorough review of the changing situation among Japanese children, published in the *American Journal of Clinical Nutrition* (2000), Dr. Mitsunori Murata of Tokyo Women's Medical College also noted that about 80 percent of all students in junior and senior high school have developed a sedentary lifestyle outside school. This, of course, only compounds the issue. Given these changes, the upward trend in the incidence of cardiovascular disease in Japanese cities is not entirely surprising. Men of all ages and older women have seen significant gains in body weight and a higher BMI over the last decade. In contrast, young to middle-aged women living in Japan's largest cities have actually seen a decrease in BMI over the last twenty-five years, most likely due to the tremendous social pressure for young Japanese women to remain thin.

In an attempt to provide guidance to the public, Japan's Ministry of Health, Labour, and Welfare unveiled the new Japanese Food Guide Spinning Top in 2005. It is presented here, and as you can see, it is actually quite brilliant in its design. Physical activity and exercise drive the spinning of the top, and without it, the top will fall over. It is also clear that should any dietary segment of the spinning top be over- or underconsumed, complete balance will be lost—the spinning top will topple and brain health will be compromised.

There is no question that hormones can influence our mood and our behaviors and there are a number of studies showing that the Western diet increases androgens (male hormones including testosterone). As long ago as 1979, researchers showed that switching from a traditional South African diet to a typical North American diet increased androgen levels. A recent study by Dr. Christina Wang and colleagues from UCLA showed that reducing dietary fat and increasing dietary fiber lowered circulating androgen levels by 12 percent in healthy middle-aged men. The animal fat appears to be the issue rather than meat per se, because separate research using fatty meat, tofu, and lean meat showed that only *fatty* meat caused significant post-meal increases in testosterone.

While testosterone obviously has its place in a healthy body, too much appears to negatively influence the brain. Researchers from the National Institute on Aging have shown, in the journal *Neurobiology of Aging* (2005), that elderly men with the highest testosterone levels are at the highest risk for cerebral atrophy (withering of brain cells). This means that the male hormone, in high levels, may actually be shrinking the brain. When it comes to behavior, high testosterone has a well-established link to aggression in humans and animals.

A number of studies have shown that adults guilty of violent crimes have higher testosterone levels than those who commit nonviolent crimes. Incarcerated adults who break the rules in correction facilities are more likely to have high testosterone levels. In a sample of almost 4,500 U.S. soldiers, higher testosterone levels were associated with job difficulties, antisocial behavior, marital difficulties, drug and alcohol abuse, and violent acts. Individuals with a background of aggressiveness, impulsive behaviors, and suicide attempts have higher levels of testosterone inside the fluid surrounding the central nervous system. In children, aggressiveness and antisocial behavior have been associated with higher testosterone and other androgens including dehydroepiandrosterone (DHEA). Remember that interesting new study we talked about in the journal *Nutrition* showing that those who attempt suicide have a much lower intake of dietary fiber than those who do not. Is it possible that dietary fiber could lower the risk of suicide by providing foods rich in nutrients, and by modestly lowering the male hormone associated with suicide attempts? Maybe so.

Experimentally, chronic testosterone administration lowers serotonin levels in the brain. The combination of low serotonin and elevated testosterone may set the stage for the literal one-two punch of impulsivity and aggression. It is entirely possible that the changing Japanese diet is bringing with it changes in androgen levels, which in turn are influencing brain and behavior. Components of the traditional diet have been shown to keep testosterone in check. Green tea, soy, fiber, and fish oils have all been shown to moderately lower blood testosterone levels. Incredibly, maternal intake of these food items during pregnancy may have long-term consequences on hormonal levels years later in the child. The influences of dietary intake on behavior may therefore become established in pregnancy and early life.

Despite the alarming dietary changes, the possible brain and behavior consequences have global relativity. As you can see from the comparative graphs, the Japanese are still way behind North Americans when it comes to animal fat, sugar, vegetable oil, meat, etc., and way ahead when it comes to fish and seafood. The effects of green tea, ginger, seaweeds, fermented soy, and other phytonutrients may also have added protective value. The Japanese still experience much lower rates of cardiovascular disease and many cancers and brain-related illnesses than North Americans do. They also enjoy the greatest longevity on earth. As for the rises in violent crime and antisocial behavior, these are of course alarming for Japan, but on a global scale it is still an extremely safe place to live and visit. Japan's crime rates are extremely low by North American standards: homicide is eleven times lower than in the United States, serious assaults are twenty-three times lower, and robbery/violent thefts are sixty-three times lower.

Fast food and Western influences aside, the traditional Japanese diet is all about presentation, variety, and the experience of dining itself. In a recent study published in the journal *Appetite* (2005), researchers from Kyoto University showed that a nutritionally balanced diet, with plenty of vegetables and variety, was held as the most important attribute of "healthy eating" among the Japanese. A large percentage of Japanese rated enjoying eating with family and friends and swallowing after sufficient *chewing* as "extremely important" in healthy eating. Having food with family and friends can make the experience of eating more enjoyable, and is certainly better than watching TV or playing videogames while eating.

But what about chewing your food, isn't that an old folk tale? The answer is absolutely not. Beyond the obvious assistance in digestion chewing provides, there are even more interesting brain connections emerging from research on mastication (chewing). In the last few years, a number of studies have shown that chewing increases blood flow to many of the brain's regions. An increase in blood flow to the areas involved in mastication would be expected, but what emerges is that chewing increases widespread blood flow to brain, an increase that's not due to jaw movement itself. Chewing increases blood flow by 10 to 28 percent in many regions. Let's keep in the back of our minds that many brain-related conditions, from Alzheimer's to depression, involve subpar blood flow to various brain regions. Let's also remember that nerve cells are now known to generate in adulthood and that nutrition, exercise, and an enriched environment can influence childhood and adult nerve generation.

In a recent study in *NeuroReport* (2005), Japanese researchers showed that the act of chewing can positively influence the survival of newly generated adult brain cells. Soft food, which requires little chewing effort, *reduced* the survival of the newly generated brain cells. In an animal study in *Brain Research* (2001), researchers from Tokyo Dental College showed that soft foods in early life actually impaired cognitive function and learning later in adulthood. The act of chewing has also been shown to reduce stress and stimulate the activity of GABA receptors, the same receptors acted upon by anti-anxiety medications. A number of recent studies have also shown that chewing gum improves memory, attention, and cognitive function in healthy adults. Finally, research shows that the loss of many teeth and impaired mastication in adulthood is associated with an increased risk of dementia.

Obviously, eating a donut and drinking a soda require minimal mastication compared to a high-fiber bowl of granola or salad with nuts and apples. As reported in *Japan Now* (July/August 1999), dietician Asako Aramaki found that the Japanese who hold on to the chopstick diet have a more nutritionally healthy diet, more balanced blood sugar, and less nutrient deficiencies than those who do not eat with chopsticks. Eating with chopsticks is traditionally associated with a slower, more methodical consumption of a meal, one that involves more chewing and less "wolfing down" food. When you eat slowly, the brain picks up the signal that you are full long before a bunch of extra calories have been consumed. Fast food is not only served quickly, it is packaged to be easily and rapidly consumed. In words that would make any soothsayer proud, Rolf Kreiner, then McDonald's director of marketing for West Germany, stated in *Time* magazine September 17, 1973, "We are educating people to a whole new way of life—eating with your fingers instead of forks," and they clearly succeeded in that mission.

In a study presented at the North American Association for the Study of Obesity's Annual Scientific Meeting in Vancouver (2005), researchers from the University of Liverpool showed that chewing gum helps to curb appetite and the desire for sweet snacks in the afternoon. At the same obesity conference, researchers from Nagoya University, Japan, showed that chewing less and eating fast may lead to obesity in adults. They looked at almost 3,500 men and women, and even after controlling for total calorie intake and various lifestyle factors, eating meals more rapidly was associated with a significantly larger BMI.

Japanese food has become more popular in the last decade or so in North America, particularly in major metropolitan areas where there are sizable Japanese communities. Traditional Japanese food is consumed in the most natural way possible. For maximum flavor and nutrient value, fish is often eaten raw and vegetables are minimally cooked. Until recent years, most Japanese kitchens didn't even have conventional ovens, and even though most households now have an oven, they are not used to the same degree as in Western cooking. The end result is greater consumption of foods that are steamed, boiled, sautéed, or stir-fried on low heat versus long cooking times in dry heat ovens. As you'll recall from chapter 2, avoiding overcooked foods in dry heat will greatly reduce your intake of AGEs, which promote inflammation and oxidative stress.

Traditional Japanese meals are the opposite of super-sized when it comes to portions—however, they are not minimized when it comes to variety. The traditional meal is made up of several small dishes at one sitting; it is not uncommon to have six or seven different small plates and bowls in front of you while dining, each one comprised of many different food components. A recent survey showed that older Japanese women consume more than one hundred different types of food per week! The typical Western food consumer is doing well if they hit thirty types. We have talked about the protection of dietary synergy, how antioxidants work together, and obviously the greater the variety of foods, the more opportunity for synergy in brain protection. In my experiences of traditional home cooking in Japan, I have been amazed at how many bowls and small plates (with wide nutritional variety) can be squeezed onto the tables in Japanese homes—not a square centimeter is spared.

The traditional Japanese breakfast is worth describing because it is the polar opposite of a sugary drink and a donut. While there are regional differences, the typical Japanese breakfast includes miso soup, rice, pickled vegetables, a thick omelet cube, and grilled fish (e.g., salmon). I know this sounds like a lot of work for today's working couples, but the importance of a solid breakfast is worth underscoring. Many North American adults and children forgo breakfast altogether, and this is not without brain and behavioral consequences. Between 1965 and 1991, breakfast consumption in North American kids (preschool to early teens) has declined by up to 20 percent depending on age. For late teens (fifteen to eighteen), skipping breakfast has dropped by 30 percent. But 59 percent of high school students skip four or more times per week, 21 percent of eight- and nine-year-olds do not eat breakfast every day, and 42 percent of twelve- and thirteen-year-olds do not eat breakfast every day. While far more Japanese children do eat breakfast compared to their North American counterparts, an increasing number are now skipping breakfast, according to research by Mitsunori Murata of Tokyo Women's Medical College.

Eating breakfast is a habit, and children start to experience a drop in quality of life when they fall away from regular breakfast consumption. We have discussed the growing sleep debt among our youth, and research shows that children and teens who sleep less are more likely to forgo breakfast as they try to get out of the house on time. This combined lack of sleep and low brain fuel is a disaster for mental sharpness and mood, and it sets the stage for an increase in stress hormones and an overconsumption of calories later in the day. Research shows that in tweens and teens followed over ten years, those eating a morning cereal breakfast weigh less than peers who do not eat cereal in the morning. In addition to not overconsuming more calories later in the day, the link between breakfast and protection against weight gain may have to do with the calcium that comes along with the milk, the fiber in whole grains, and that cereal displaces other items high in saturated fat.

When it comes to brain function, breakfast may be the most important meal of the day, for children and adults alike. Research shows that breakfast enhances cognitive and academic performance, with the effects particularly pronounced in the areas of memory recall and longer-term memory. The effects of breakfast on memory function have been noted for several hours after.

International studies also show that breakfast consumption benefits

Japanese college students who report higher levels of fatigue are more
likely to . . .

1. Skip breakfast
2. Snack between meals
3. Consume single-item meals
4. Eat more instant foods
5. Eat more confectionary
6. Eat meals at irregular times
7. Eat meals with no vegetables
8. Eat meals with no fruits

overall grades, school attendance, and even punctuality. Of real interest
to me are the handful of studies showing that breakfast consumption
improves outcomes in the psychological realm. In one study, beneficial
changes in childhood depression and hyperactivity were noted with
increased school breakfast adherence. A separate study showed that when
breakfast consumption increased nutritional status, there were improvements in psychosocial functioning. Additional research published in the
journal *Appetite* (2003) and the *International Journal of Food Science and
Nutrition* (1997) shows that breakfast consumption in children promotes
positive mood, alertness, and contentment.

A fiber-containing breakfast appears to be the way to go when it
comes to pronounced effects on mood and combating fatigue. Researchers
from Tufts University recently published a study in the journal *Physiology
and Behavior* (2005) that showed that an oatmeal breakfast was far better
in improving cognitive performance in nine- to eleven-year-olds than was
a ready-to-eat cereal with lower fiber and protein and more sugar. In an
article in the *International Journal of Obesity* (2003), researchers from the
Netherlands showed that, compared to a simple carbohydrate breakfast, a
complex carbohydrate (three times more fiber) was associated with lower
fatigue scores and a higher degree of satiety. Dr. Andrew Smith and colleagues from Cardiff University, U.K., found that high-fiber (15 percent or
more) cereals versus low-fiber (3 percent) breakfast cereals seem to have a
fatigue-reducing affect. Dr. Smith's study, published in the journal *Appetite*
(2001), showed that high-fiber breakfasts are associated with decreased

fatigue, emotional distress, and cognitive difficulties. The emotional distress connection is very, very interesting, because recent work from Dr. Smith in *Nutritional Neuroscience* (2002) shows that regular consumption of breakfast cereal is associated with lower levels of the stress hormone cortisol.

While the traditional Japanese diet is a nutritional powerhouse that promotes brain function and provides much needed nutrients, a good old bowl of high-fiber, low-sugar cereal is also a great way to get the day started when time is tight. I'm not talking about a bowl of granulated sugar with some vitamins and minerals added. The cereal to choose is low-sugar and inclusive of whole grain. Check the fiber content on the label and compare it to other cereals.

Before moving on to the recipes, I will leave you with one more study on the importance of breakfast and, more specifically, breakfast quality. Dr. Claire Pincock of Reading University, U.K., and colleagues published important research in the journal *Appetite* (2003). The study showed just how bad our current sugary breakfast snacks are. They found that eating cereal rich in fibrous complex carbohydrates, compared to consuming a sugar-based drink, helped to maintain attention and memory throughout the morning in nine- to sixteen-year-olds. The children consumed the breakfast at about 8:00 a.m., and were followed up every hour after until 12:00 noon. The whole-grain cereal helped prevent the normal downward slide in mental performance as the time ticked toward lunch hour. Based on everything we have just discussed, this seems reasonable. But what was shocking was that in the sugar-drink breakfast group, the participants demonstrated, in some realms, the cognitive performances of seventy-year-olds!

Summary

The sharp rises in brain-related conditions, depression, behavioral problems, and violence have been cause for great concern in Japan. This recent increase of brain-related conditions has been occurring hand in hand with the disappearance of the traditional Japanese diet. In particular, Japanese youth are turning toward a Western fast food–oriented diet, and their dietary choices appear to be having behavioral and mood-related consequences. The alarming trends in Japan are an urgent call for us to take a look at nutritional influences on brain health from a societal perspective.

Almost thirty years ago, key aspects of the Okinawan diet and the incredible longevity of these Japanese people were introduced to the West by Dr. Yasuo Kagawa. However, there was no way of knowing that in a very short period of time, Okinawans would rapidly succumb to the lure of the American-packaged taste of salt, sugar, and saturated fat. Fast food has been like a slow-acting smallpox epidemic carried by foreigners into the region. The results have been devastating.

Thankfully, the Japanese diet still contains items with tremendous protective properties in brain health. Green tea, ginger, fermented soy, fish and seafood, sesame, seaweed, and a variety of colorful phytonutrients continue to be consumed in significant quantities in today's Japanese diet relative to the West. These dietary items contain nutrients that can influence brain health and behavior through direct nerve-cell protecting properties, and also indirectly by influencing brain chemicals and hormones that have been tied to mood and aggression.

In Japan, the traditional diet has placed a strong emphasis on a solid and nutritious breakfast. New research highlights just how important breakfast is in firing up the brain to run on all cylinders throughout the day. A nutritious breakfast improves mental function and focus, keeps stress hormones in check, and maintains energy levels, all of which translates into better academic performance in school and cognitive function in the workplace. Improved mental focus, through a solid breakfast, also translates into improved behavior in school settings. Given the wealth of research, a nutritious breakfast might be one place to start when trying to remedy the behavioral problems encroaching into North American and Japanese schools. Sadly, more and more North American and Japanese children are skipping breakfast, and yet a bowl of fiber-rich, low-sugar cereal or oatmeal is probably the simplest way to ensure a child is functioning in top gear.

Brain Diet Samplers

The following are some meal ideas to promote your brain health. I am deeply grateful to nutrition consultant Yoshiko Sato of Tokyo, Japan, who helped to infuse a Japanese flavor into some of the meals. Hopefully they will give you an idea of how easy and delicious it can be to both fuel and protect your brain. Meals are suitable for four. Many of the dishes involve a light sauté—remember that deep-frying foods, using processed foods, and using long cooking time on high, dry heat will maximize the production of the AGEs we discussed earlier. Some of these meals involve broiling. Enjoy some meals on the broiler, but it is best not make them an everyday event. When it comes to cooking with olive oil, extra virgin is loaded with antioxidants, but it must be kept in a dark bottle in a dark place in your home. Research shows that oil stored in clear plastic bottles under supermarket light will lose at least 30 percent of important antioxidants. The Japanese flavor and antioxidant/anti-inflammatory spices found in some of the meals are for obvious brain-healthy reasons. Enjoy!

RICE PAPER ROLLS

8   sheets of 12-inch round rice paper
16   medium/large shrimp, cooked, peeled, deveined
1½   cups red cabbage or red lettuce, shredded
2   small radishes, cut to thin circular slices
1   small carrot, shredded
½   cup cilantro
1   small avocado, skinned and cut to small wedges, sprinkled with lemon juice
8   tablespoons of ginger-peanut dipping sauce (e.g. The Ginger People®)

Add warm to hot water (comfortable to hands) to a large glass cooking bowl. Immerse one sheet of rice paper in water for 10 seconds and lay on a clean, dampened dish towel. Gently wrap ingredients (except dipping sauce!) into rice paper, allowing that there will be a total of 8 rolls. Each roll should be neatly wrapped aproximately 6 inches long and 1 to 2 inches wide. Cut if desired. Use ginger-peanut dipping sauce.

ROASTED RED PEPPER SOUP

3   large roasted red bell peppers, skin, seeds removed after roasting, cut to wedges
2   cups tomato juice
1   clove garlic
1½   cups vegetable stock (e.g. Imagine brand Organic)
1   tablespoon olive oil
¼   teaspoon cumin

Pinch cayenne pepper

Sea salt, black pepper to taste

In food processor or large blender combine tomato juice, bell peppers, and garlic and purée. Transfer to large cooking pot and add stock and remaining ingredients. Simmer on very low heat for 15 to 20 minutes. Garnish with fresh chopped parsley and nuts of choice.

PURPLE-POWER SALAD

½   red apple, cut into thin wedges with skin on

1   medium purple onion, sliced

2   cups purple cauliflower

2   tablespoons parsley, medium chopped

In a large pot boil cauliflower for about 5 minutes or less to maintain crispness. Drain and refrigerate. Add sliced onion and apples to separate bowls of water and steep for a few minutes. The water for the apple should be lightly salted. Mix all ingredients together in a large salad bowl. Add your favorite dressing.

WILD EDAMAME SALAD

1   cup wild rice (e.g. Riceselect™ Texmati Blend)

4   tablespoons rice vinegar

2   teaspoons honey

1   teaspoon lemon juice

2   tablespoons olive oil

     Sea salt and black pepper to taste

1   small carrot, finely chopped

½   orange bell pepper, finely chopped

½   cucumber, finely chopped

24   small shrimp, cooked, shelled, and deveined

½   cup frozen edamame (soy) beans shells removed (e.g., Cascadian Farms)

1   green onion, chopped

Cook wild rice in lightly salted water according to package directions and let cool. In a large salad bowl combine rice vinegar, honey, lemon juice, olive oil, salt, and pepper. Add cooled wild rice, and then combine vegetables, shrimp, and finally edamame. Garnish with green onion.

DOUBLE WILD SALMON AND RICE

1   teaspoon canola oil
4   fillets wild salmon
    Sea salt and black pepper to taste
1½ teaspoons fresh ginger, finely chopped
1½ teaspoons fresh garlic, finely chopped
2   teaspoons low-sodium soy sauce
12 large asparagus spears
1   cup wild rice (e.g. Riceselect™ Texmati Blend)

In large skillet heat the canola oil. Place salmon on skillet skin side down
and sprinkle on salt and pepper. Sauté until cooked through (about 5 to 6
minutes) on both sides. Remove from pan and sauté ginger and garlic in the
remaining oil until color changes. Turn off heat to skillet and add soy sauce
and mix into the garlic and ginger for just about 10 to 15 seconds. Add soy-
ginger-garlic mixture to the top of salmon fillets. Add lemon juice if desired.
Serve with steamed asparagus (5 to 7 minutes), and wild rice prepared as
per package directions.

GREEN TEA SOBA SALAD

½   pound extra firm tofu, drained and cut into 1-inch
    cubes
1   tablespoon canola oil
4   ounces fresh string beans, ends removed and cut to
    thirds
1   pound green tea soba noodles
3   tablespoons olive oil
12 cherry tomatoes, halved
1   tablespoon black sesame seeds
    Sea salt and black pepper to taste

In a heated skillet sauté tofu cubes in canola oil to golden color and set
aside. Sauté cut string beans to desired firmness and set aside with tofu in
refrigerator to cool down. In a large pot, boil green tea soba for 6 to 7 minutes or to desired firmness, stirring occasionally. Drain soba and rinse with
cold water, then add to large salad bowl and mix olive oil over the noodles.
Add tofu, beans, tomatoes, sesame seeds, salt, and pepper.

KABOCHA—JAPANESE PUMPKIN SOUP

½   medium onion, sliced
1   tablespoon canola oil
¾   pound Kabocha pumpkin (or acorn squash), skin and
    seeds removed, cut into medium cubes

1   cup vegetable stock (e.g. Imagine Organic)

1½ cups water

½   pound soft or silken tofu, drained

½   cup rice milk (e.g. Rice Dream™)
    Sea salt and black pepper to taste

In a large heated pot, slightly brown onion in the canola oil. Add Kabocha (or acorn squash), vegetable stock, and water. Cook for about 7 minutes, stirring occasionally. Transfer Kabocha to large blender, add tofu, and puree until smooth. Return blended ingredients to pot on very low heat. Add rice milk, sea salt, and black pepper to taste. Ready in just a few minutes. Garnish with parsley.

DAIKON AND CARROT PICKLE

1½ cups daikon, shredded

½   cup shredded carrots

½   teaspoon sea salt

2   tablespoons brown sugar

⅓   cup rice vinegar

1½ tablespoons white sesame seeds

In a large bowl combine daikon and carrot, and mix in salt. In a mixing bowl combine brown sugar and rice vinegar, and stir until sugar dissolves. Add to carrot and daikon mixture. Cover and chill 2 to 3 hours. Sprinkle with sesame seeds prior to serving.

OVEN-BAKED SWEET POTATO WEDGES

6   medium/large sweet potatoes

3   tablespoons canola oil

¼   teaspoon garlic powder

¼   teaspoon paprika

⅛   teaspoon cayenne pepper
    Salt and pepper to taste

Preheat oven to 420°F. Spray a baking dish or sheet with canola oil cooking spray. Cut sweet potatoes into wedges or steak fries. Mix potatoes in a large bowl with oil and spices until they are evenly coated. Add salt and pepper to taste. Place in prepared baking dish or sheet. Bake for 12 to 15 minutes and turn potatoes over, then bake for another 12 to 15 minutes, or until golden color appears.

RED AND BLACK BEAN SALAD

⅛   teaspoon cumin powder
⅛   teaspoon garam masala
⅛   teaspoon turmeric
3   tablespoons olive oil
1   can black beans, drained and rinsed
1   can red beans, drained and rinsed
2   green onions, chopped
½   small purple onion, finely chopped
8   cherry tomatoes, halved
½   cup chopped cilantro
1   red bell pepper, medium chopped
2   tablespoons lime juice

In a skillet heat cumin, garam masala, and turmeric in 1 tablespoon olive oil. In a large salad bowl combine the beans, onions, tomatoes, cilantro, and bell pepper. Combine the remaining 2 tablespoons of olive oil with the spices and lime juice, then mix into salad. Serve on Romaine lettuce.

SARDINE PASTA BRAIN-BOOSTER

1   box whole wheat penne pasta (e.g. Ronzoni Healthy Harvest™)
3   tablespoons olive oil
½   medium red bell pepper, finely chopped
3   cloves garlic, finely chopped
2   cans sardines in tomato sauce
    Romano cheese for garnish

Boil pasta in a large pot to desired firmness. In a skillet heat 2 tablespoons olive oil and sauté the red pepper and ever-so-slightly brown the garlic. Add the sardines and tomato sauce and warm through. Drain the pasta and toss the pasta with 1 tablespoon of olive oil. Add the sardines and tomato sauce mixture, then garnish with chopped parsley and a small amount of Romano cheese.

TURMERIC RICE

2   cups vegetable stock (e.g. Imagine Organic Broth)
1   cup brown basmati rice (e.g. Lundberg California brown)
1   tablespoon rice bran oil
1   teaspoon turmeric powder
1   pinch cayenne pepper

1   tablespoon raisins

Bring the vegetable stock to boil in a pot, add rice and remaining ingredients except for raisins. Cover tightly and simmer on low heat for about 50 minutes. Remove from heat and keep covered for 10 minutes. Stir when finished and add raisins.

ANCHOVY IQ SALAD

2   heads romaine lettuce, leaves quartered
3   cups spinach leaves
½   pound fresh mozzarella, cut into small segments
12 cherry tomatoes, halved
1   can of anchovies in olive oil (with or without capers)

In extra large salad bowl, combine lettuce, spinach, cherry tomatoes, and mozzarella cheese. Place anchovies on top with olive oil. Add lemon juice and black pepper to taste.

BLACK SESAME SALMON

4   salmon fillets
    Sea salt and black pepper to taste
4   pinches garlic powder
4   tablespoons whole wheat or brown rice flour
2   egg whites
6   tablespoons black and white sesame seeds
3   tablespoons canola oil

Remove salmon skin, sprinkle salt and pepper on both sides of fillet and a pinch of garlic powder on each. Place flour on plate and pat a thin layer onto both sides of salmon. Place the egg whites in a small bowl and brush the whites onto the salmon. Spread sesame seeds on a separate plate and pat both sides of the salmon onto the seeds. In a skillet heat the oil and cook until white seeds are golden brown and salmon is cooked through. Garnish with cilantro and use lemon if desired.

TURKEY OR CHICKEN MEATBALL SOUP

2   tablespoons olive oil
3   cloves garlic, finely chopped
½   small onion, finely chopped
1   pound ground turkey or chicken
½   cup whole wheat bread crumbs
1   tablespoon fresh parsley
¼   teaspoon garlic powder

1   egg, beaten
½ tablespoon ketchup
2   cups vegetable stock (e.g., Imagine Organic)
2   cups water

In a skillet heat the olive oil and sauté the garlic and onion for less than one minute—to the earliest signs of browning. In a large bowl, combine the garlic and onion with the turkey or chicken, bread crumbs, parsley, garlic powder, egg, and ketchup. Form into meatballs. Place mixure in a stockpot and add the prepared vegetable stock and water; boil for 10 to 15 minutes, or until cooked through. Serve with 8 ounces separately cooked whole wheat or brown rice noodles in the soup.

SWEET POTATO CARROT SOUP

1   tablespoon canola oil
½ teaspoon garam masala
¼ teaspoon turmeric
¼ teaspoon cumin powder
1   teaspoon finely chopped ginger
1   small onion, chopped
1   garlic clove, chopped
3   cups vegetable broth (e.g. Imagine Organic)
2   large carrots, chopped
1   large sweet potato, washed and cut into chunks with skin on
    Sea salt and pepper to taste

In a large pot heat oil, spices, onion, and garlic until golden. Add vegetable broth, carrots, and sweet potato. Bring to a boil, then cover and simmer on very low heat for 45 minutes to 1 hour. Transfer to large blender and purée, or use handheld blender. Add sea salt and pepper to taste.

BUFFALO OMEGA-3 BURGERS

1½ pounds ground buffalo meat
½ small onion, finely chopped
1   tablespoon parsley, finely chopped
1   tablespoon Worcestershire sauce
1   tablespoon ketchup
1   small hot chili pepper or jalapeño pepper, finely chopped (optional)
3   tablespoons whole wheat bread crumbs
1   tablespoon ground pecans

In a mixing bowl combine all ingredients and shape into patties of desired size. Cook on a nonstick skillet for about 7 to 10 minutes or to desired doneness. Remember that buffalo meat is lower in fat and will dry out quickly if overcooked.

TANDOORI CHICKEN

4   chicken breasts (6 ounces each) skin removed, cut into
     1½-inch cubes
1   teaspoon garam masala
1   teaspoon ginger powder
1   teaspoon turmeric
1   teaspoon cayenne pepper
2   cloves crushed garlic
1   6-ounce container plain, fat-free yogurt
     Sea salt to taste

With a sharp knife, cut about halfway into the chicken breast or use a fork to puncture holes. In a large bowl mix all the remaining ingredients and add the chicken. Refrigerate, covered, for at least 12 hours. Use a roasting rack, and cook at 400°F for about 30 to 35 minutes or grill for 10 to 12 minutes.

WASABI SALMON BURGER

2   cans boneless wild pink salmon, drained
1   egg, beaten
½   small onion
1   teaspoon parsley flakes
¼   tablespoon finely chopped red bell pepper
½   cup whole wheat bread crumbs
1   tablespoon canola oil mayonnaise
2   pinches garlic powder
     Sea salt and black pepper to taste
2   tablespoons olive oil

In a large mixing bowl combine ingredients except for olive oil and shape into patties of desired size. Heat the skillet, add the olive oil, and heat the burgers on medium heat for a few minutes on each side. Keep in mind that while the fish has been cooked, the egg requires appropriate heat. Serve on whole wheat buns with romaine lettuce. Mix ¼ teaspoon wasabi paste from tube with an additional tablespoon of canola oil mayonnaise for a nicely spiced dressing to be divided between the burgers.

CILANTRO RICE

2   tablespoons canola oil
1   small onion, finely chopped
2   cloves garlic, finely chopped
1½   tablespoons cilantro, finely chopped
¼   teaspoon cumin
     Pinch turmeric
1   cup short grain brown rice

Heat the oil in a skillet and sauté the onion and garlic until slightly brown. Mix in the spices and heat for about 15 to 20 seconds. Add this mixture to the lightly salted boiling water and brown rice and cook as per rice package directions.

SPINACH WITH SESAME DRESSING

3   tablespoons black sesame seeds, ground
1½   tablespoons brown sugar
1   tablespoon Dashi stock (Japanese seaweed and
     mushroom broth)
3   tablespoons low-sodium soy sauce
14   ounces fresh spinach, blanched until just tender,
     chopped

In a medium bowl combine ground sesame seeds, brown sugar, and soy sauce and mix together with Dashi stock. In a large salad bowl add dressing to spinach and thoroughly mix.

SPICE FOR HEALTH CURRY

2   teaspoons Smart Balance Omega Plus Spread
1   tablespoon garlic, finely chopped
1   tablespoon ginger, finely chopped
1   large onion, finely chopped
1   pound ground chicken
2   medium carrots, finely chopped
1   medium red bell pepper, finely chopped
1¼   cups chicken stock (e.g. Imagine® Organic)
½   cup green peas
18   ounces canned whole peeled tomatoes
1   tablespoon curry powder
¼   teaspoon garam masala
1   tablespoon plain yogurt
     Salt and pepper to taste

In a hot skillet heat the Omega Plus Spread and lightly brown the garlic, ginger. and onion. Add ground chicken, carrots, and red peppers, and cook through. Add chicken stock, green peas, and whole tomatoes, and bring to near boil. Add curry powder, garam masala, yogurt, and salt and pepper to taste, and mix thoroughly. Continue to heat until desired consistency. Serve with whole wheat wraps.

EGGPLANT MISO SOUP—NO MSG

2	cups water
3	tablespoons no-MSG miso paste (e.g. Honzukuri)
1	cup Japanese eggplant, cut into strips
2	green onions, chopped
¼	teaspoon low-sodium soy sauce

In a medium pot bring water to a boil and add miso paste, stirring until dissolved. Add eggplant and green onions and cook for 5 to 7 minutes. Turn off heat and stir in soy sauce just before serving.

JAPANESE CRAB AND SEAWEED SALAD

4	tablespoons rice vinegar
2	tablespoons low-sodium soy sauce
2	tablespoons brown sugar
3	Japanese cucumbers, cut lengthwise and seeds removed
	Salt to taste
1	tablespoon dry wakame seaweed flakes (e.g. Eden Wakame Flakes)
1	6-ounce can crab meat

Combine vinegar, soy sauce, and brown sugar in small bowl and mix. Shred cucumber, place it into a medium bowl, cover with water, and add a couple of pinches of salt. Let stand for about 10 minutes and then drain well. Soak wakame in hot water according to directions, drain, and add to cucumber and crab in a large salad bowl. Blend in vinegar dressing.

CHICKEN-SHITAKE STIR FRY

2	tablespoons canola oil
4	free-range chicken breasts, cut to strips
1	tablespoon ginger, finely chopped
1	tablespoon garlic, finely chopped
2	cups broccoli crowns
3	cups bok choy
8	fresh shitake mushrooms, root tip removed and then chopped

1   small red bell pepper, medium chopped
1   red hot chili or jalapeño pepper, finely chopped
    (optional)
½   cup chicken broth (e.g., Imagine Organic)
2   tablespoons low-sodium soy sauce
1   teaspoon cornstarch
1   teaspoon sesame oil

In a large skillet or wok, heat 1 tablespoon of canola oil and cook the chicken for about 5 minutes and remove. Set aside. Add 1 tablespoon of canola oil to wok and sauté the ginger and garlic for about a minute. Add broccoli, bok choy, shitake, and peppers, and stir fry for about 5 minutes or desired cooking time. Return chicken to wok and add chicken stock. Add soy sauce and cornstarch to thicken. Mix thoroughly for about a minute. Add sesame oil and stir in. Serve with brown rice.

JAPANESE INFUSION SMOOTHIE FOR TWO
½   cup low-fat vanilla frozen yogurt
1   cup frozen blueberries
1   teaspoon ground black sesame seeds
½   teaspoon matcha green tea
1½ cups of rice milk (e.g., Rice Dream™)
2   ice cubes

In a blender combine all ingredients. Blend on high and enjoy.

ACAI MATCHA SMOOTHIE FOR TWO
1   cup rice milk (e.g., Rice Dream™)
1   cup soy milk
1   cup frozen blueberries
1   package frozen acai (e.g., Sambazon™)
2   tablespoons plain, fat-free yogurt
¼   teaspoon matcha green tea
2   ice cubes

In a blender combine all ingredients. Blend on high and enjoy.

BLACK SESAME DELIGHT FOR TWO
12 ounces plain low-fat yogurt
1/2 banana, thinly sliced
2   teaspoons black sesame paste or ground black sesame
    seeds

Combine yogurt and banana pieces in a bowl. Fold in sesame paste with a spoon. Serve cold.

10

The Brain Diet Plan:
In Health and in Sickness

The human brain is a sophisticated, yet delicate, organ. Proper development and maintenance requires a steady supply of essential nutrients. For top performance and prevention of illness, your brain needs high-grade fuel. Depending upon individual susceptibilities, brain function can be compromised when essential nutrients are taken in excess, or at inadequate levels. In this chapter, we will examine various neurological and psychiatric disorders and highlight some incredible research findings that underscore the nutritional influences on brain health.

It really is shocking how many nutrients are tied in with alterations in psychiatric and neurological conditions. Most medical doctors are unaware of this research because they have little or no training in nutrition while in medical school. This sets a tone: if it isn't discussed, how important could it really be? This information is not mystical thinking, it is not placing a crystal around your neck or some other alternative medicine babble; it is based on scientific reporting. The clear message is that many patients with psychiatric and neurological conditions do have serious nutritional issues—important enough that they require an action plan.

The Brain Diet Action Plan

- Consume a minimum of five servings of deeply colored fruits and vegetables. Choose at least one serving from the high ORAC list (chapter 2).

- Include fish at least three times per week and choose oily fish (or take a fish oil supplement). Limit or cut back on red meat to a maximum of once per week.

- Choose complex carbohydrates and avoid simple sugars. Consider brown rice, whole wheat pasta, whole grain cereals, and whole grain breads instead of white, refined, and bleached counterparts.

- Limit corn, safflower, sunflower, and soybean oils. Cook with canola oil if using high heat, and use extra virgin olive oil for a light sauté or dipping. Sesame oil is an excellent choice for salads and light cooking. Rice bran and extra virgin olive oils are filled with antioxidant phytochemicals. Avoid margarine and butter. If whole grain breads feel lonely and need some fat, dip them in a little olive oil for flavor and for some additional brain-protecting antioxidants.

- Limit intake of high AGE foods (fatty meats cooked on high heat, full-fat cheeses, highly processed foods, dry baked goods cooked on high heat). These foods promote oxidative stress and inflammation and compromise brain function. The general rule is that AGE is limited with lower cooking temperature, less cooking time, and in the presence of moisture.

- Include anti-inflammatory and antioxidant culinary spices, herbs, and moderate teas and coffee (decaffeinated if you are bothered by caffeine).

- Take a daily multivitamin.

Whether you are trying to improve your day-to-day brain functioning, prevent the onset of a brain-related condition, or reduce the symptoms of certain brain conditions, these are the seven universal steps to live by. The Brain Diet plan is based on thousands of scientific studies that show, beyond any doubt, that the human brain needs premium fuel. The brain is delicate, and it is also resilient. It can "get by" for years and years on subpar nutrition; however, it will always be sluggish and operate below top cognitive performance. Simply getting by is not enough if you want to stay at the top of your game, not only in the here and now but years into the future as well. The nutritional choices you make every day become routine—the reality is that dietary decisions are powerful decisions that can affect brain performance a few hours and a few decades

Wheat Alternatives:	Amaranth	Kasha	Quinoa	Rye
	Barley	Millet	Rice	Tapioca
	Buckwheat	Oats		

Dairy Alternatives: Soy beverages/cheeses/yogurts
Rice beverages/cheeses/yogurts
Almond beverages
Oat beverages
Note: In considering a milk alternative, choose
beverages fortified with calcium, vitamins A&D
and vitamin B12.

later. Oxidative stress and inflammation are characteristic of virtually all the brain conditions to be discussed in the following pages. Food sensitivities/intolerances may also play a role in many of these conditions.

Note that the proper identification of food sensitivities requires medical guidance from a nutritionally oriented medical doctor or licensed naturopathic physician.

The seven steps of the Brain Diet plan apply universally. In addition, certain dietary interventions may be appropriate for specific neurological or psychiatric conditions. In particular, dietary supplements may be warranted as a complement to the Brain Diet plan. The daily multivitamin/mineral is essential to the plan and negates the need to take multiple supplements. As you will see, the blood levels of many vitamins and minerals are lower or useful as a preventative in most of these brain conditions. It is important to cover all nutritional bases first; essential fatty acids, beneficial bacteria (probiotics), fiber, and food-based phytonutrient antioxidants (green food supplement) should be prioritized.

As mentioned already, nutritional interventions and dietary supplements are never a substitute for appropriate mental and neurological care. If you have any medical condition, the use of dietary supplements must be disclosed to your treating physician so that the appropriateness of the supplement and any potential drug interactions can be identified.

Occasionally brand names are recommended because of my specific confidence in a select few products. For example, Genuine Health's greens+™ is the green food formula used in the groundbreaking

University of Toronto studies. Nature's Way Perika™ and Ginkgold™ utilize the specific extracts of St John's wort and ginkgo biloba, respectively, that have been used in clinical research. Concentrated eicosapentaenoic acid (EPA; o3mega+ joy™) is the only enteric-coated EPA product available and one of only a handful of fish oil products to receive the endorsement of the International Fish Oil Standards (IFOS) group, an independent watchdog body. The unique enteric-coating cuts down on the fishy repeat and aftertaste found with some brands.

Most dietary supplements should be divided as much as possible. For example, if St. John's wort and Ginkgo daily doses are 900 mg and 240 mg (respectively), such doses should be 300 mg (St. John's wort) and 80 mg (ginkgo) taken three times a day. Use of dietary supplements should always be disclosed to your health-care provider.

Brain Disorders

DEPRESSION

There are a number of formally diagnosable conditions revolving around the term depression; specific diagnosis may depend on duration and presence of coexisting symptoms. Central to depressive disorders are periods of low mood that are beyond extreme sadness; much more serious, depression often involves changes in appetite, sleep, energy, and cognitive functioning, and a loss of interest in previously pleasurable activities. Depressive disorders are common in North America, with more severe forms affecting 5 to 7 percent of the population at any given time. Over a lifetime, up to 20 percent of North Americans experience depressive disorders. The rates of depression have risen dramatically over the last century, particularly post-1945, when rates were up to twenty times lower than they are today. This serious rise in the incidence of depression has been accompanied by an earlier onset of symptoms. In other words, more of our youth are experiencing symptoms of depression than ever before. Research shows that the increase in depression is not simply a result in changes in the attitudes of health-care providers, society, or diagnostic criteria. Environmental factors play a role, and nutritional intake is now being recognized as underappreciated.

Nutritional factors have been shown to influence not only unipolar major depressive disorder, but also bipolar or manic depression, where episodes of depression alternate with periods of mania (excessive elevation in mood or euphoria). Nutrition may also affect the symptoms of seasonal affective disorder—a variant of depression that typically begins in late autumn and ends in early spring.

Depressive disorders are extremely complex and not every patient presents in exactly the same way. By the same token, not every patient will respond to the main treatment interventions—medications and psychotherapy. Both of these forms of treatment are an absolute must, and no diet or nutritional supplement should ever take the place of appropriate mental health care. Sadly, there are far too many individuals with depressive disorders who remain undiagnosed and untreated. For most of these people, appropriate therapy and/or medications are the ticket to turning the illness around.

The reality with depression, however, is that despite standard interventions, many patients remain completely treatment resistant, or do not recover to the expected degree. It is well known that many patients discontinue medications due to side effects. This is where nutritional intervention comes into play. It can be used as a means to protect against depressive symptoms, treat depressive symptoms, and augment the response to standard care.

NUTRITIONAL CONSIDERATIONS

- Fish and seafood consumption is associated with lower rates of depression, both within and between nations.
- Omega-3 fatty acids from fish, and one in particular called eicosapentaenoic acid (EPA), can improve the effectiveness of antidepressant medications.
- Countries that consume greater amounts of sugar have higher rates of depression.
- Individuals with depression consume greater amounts of carbohydrates and sugar.
- A number of studies show that patients with depression have low levels of folic acid.
- The administration of just 500 mcg of folic acid improves the effectiveness of, and lowers side effects associated with, antidepressant medications.
- Low levels of thiamine are associated with depressive symptoms.
- In at least four double-blind, placebo-controlled studies, an improvement in thiamine status is associated with improved mood.

- Low levels of vitamin B12 have been found in patients with depression.
- Higher levels of vitamin B12 predict a better treatment outcome with standard care.
- Low levels of riboflavin (vitamin B2) are associated with depressive symptoms. Supplementation with a multivitamin preparation improves mood, specifically associated with improvements in riboflavin status.
- Vitamin D improves mood during the winter months. Lack of winter sunlight leads to lower levels of vitamin D production; therefore supplementation may be worthwhile.
- A number of studies have shown that zinc levels are low in patients with depression.
- Double-blind, placebo-controlled research has shown that just 25 mg of zinc added to antidepressant medications improves treatment outcome versus antidepressant alone.
- At least five studies have shown that low selenium intake is associated with low mood states.
- Chromium supplementation has been shown to improve mood in double-blind, placebo-controlled research involving patients with depressive symptoms.
- Magnesium deficiencies have been noted in depressive disorders and, due to magnesium's influence over many brain pathways related to depression, supplementation may be valuable.

SUPPLEMENTS TO THE BRAIN DIET IN DEPRESSION
- Eicosapentaenoic acid (EPA)—1000 mg daily (as o3mega+joy™)
- 5HTP—200–300 mg daily (never mix with antidepressants)
- SAMe—800 mg daily (not for bipolar depression)
- St. John's wort—900 mg daily (as Perika™; never mix with antidepressants)
- Ginkgo biloba—240 mg daily (as Ginkgold™; most effective for depression in older persons)
- Magnesium citrate—300 mg daily

ANXIETY DISORDERS AND STRESS

Anxiety disorders are the most common type of brain condition in North America. As with depressive symptoms, anxiety occurs on a continuum from occasional stress-induced anxiety to debilitating fear and apprehension. At the debilitating end of the spectrum, there are five major anxiety disorders—panic disorder, obsessive-compulsive disorder, phobic disorders, generalized anxiety disorder, and posttraumatic stress disorder. As previously discussed, stress feeds many medical conditions, and it certainly promotes anxiety. In turn, anxiety and fear promote stress. Panic disorder is characterized by the spontaneous and unexpected onset of intense anxiety. The panic attack itself involves both physical and cognitive features. Heart palpitations, dizziness, shortness of breath, abdominal discomfort, chest pain, and other physical symptoms are often accompanied by fear of losing control or "going crazy," feelings of unreality, or fear that some sort of danger is imminent. In the case of generalized anxiety, many of these symptoms and excessive worry present on a continuous basis.

Panic attacks turn into panic disorder if they are followed by one month or more of behavioral changes or persistent fear related to more attacks. I know firsthand what it is like to have panic attacks. It is strange writing about the symptoms in medical terms because the words can never capture the sense of sheer terror that accompanies an attack.

Specific phobias involve significant and persistent fear (excessive or unreasonable) that is initiated by the presence or anticipation of an object or situation. The situation might be driving through a tunnel, riding in an elevator, flying in an airplane, or any number of other triggers. Social phobia, or social anxiety disorder, involves significant and persistent fear in social or performance situations where the individual is exposed to unfamiliar people and/or to possible scrutiny by others. Obsessive-compulsive disorder involves recurrent thoughts, impulses, and/or images that are beyond the worry of real-life problems. The thoughts, impulses, or images are extremely distressing, so much so that the individual will make efforts to suppress or neutralize them with another thought or action. For example, the individual may repeatedly wash or count in an effort to reduce the anxiety or prevent a terrible event from occurring. Posttraumatic stress disorder (PTSD) involves the experience of, or witness to, the most extreme forms of trauma. In particular, events that involve actual or threatened death, serious injury, or threat to an individual's integrity can trigger PTSD. The individual with PTSD re-experiences the event through dreams or intrusive thoughts, avoids stimuli that are (even remotely) related to the trauma, and remains in a state of hypervigilance. This hypervigilant state promotes a state of chronic stress, and it is likely the reason that those with PTSD go on to have much higher rates of physical illness. PTSD patients are prone to autoimmune conditions, inflammatory disorders, cardiovascular disease, diabetes, arthritis, psoriasis, and thyroid disease.

NUTRITIONAL CONSIDERATIONS

- Selenium deficiencies many promote anxiety.
- A low-fat diet may improve stress resistance. This effect is likely to be due to reducing inflammation-promoting saturated fats. Note that omega-3 fatty acids have been shown to reduce stress and adrenal gland activation.
- Niacin (vitamin B3) has been shown to reduce anxious and aggressive behavior in animals. Anecdotal human evidence suggests that niacinamide can be helpful in anxiety disorders.
- Chronic deficiency of thiamine may set the stage for anxious behaviors.
- Low levels of vitamin B6 may set the stage for anxiety.
- Even mild deficiencies of vitamin E may set the stage for anxious behavior.
- Mild deficiencies of vitamin C have been associated with subjective measures of anxiety.
- Case reports and animal studies suggest that omega-3 fatty acids can dampen anxiety/phobic behavior.
- Even mild deficiencies of magnesium are associated with anxiety. Case reports and animal studies suggest magnesium is helpful in dampening anxiety.
- Caffeine may promote anxiety in sensitive individuals. Coffee, tea, and other sources of caffeine should be eliminated and reintroduced slowly to determine if there is an effect on symptoms.
- Simple carbohydrates and sugar snacks should be minimized. Anxiety-prone individuals may have a worsening of symptoms when blood sugar levels quickly dip down after sugary snacks. Spiking blood glucose with nonfibrous simple sugars can elevate blood lactate. Note that lactate has been shown to induce panic in numerous studies.

SUPPLEMENTS TO THE BRAIN DIET IN ANXIETY

- Eicosapentaenoic acid (EPA)—1000 mg (as o3mega+ joy™)
- ZenBev™—1–2 tablespoons in the morning upon waking
- 5HTP—200–300 mg daily (never mix with antidepressants or St. Johns wort)
- Inositol—12 grams (research in panic disorder and OCD)

- St. John's wort—900 mg daily (as Perika™—preliminary research supports usefulness in OCD and generalized anxiety disorder; never mix with antidepressants)
- L-theanine from green tea—200 mg (as Sun brand)
- Milk protein hydrolysate—150–300 mg (choose Seriane™ or TryptoZen™)
- Magnesium citrate—300 mg
- Passionflower—300 mg (standardized to 3.5 percent isovitexin)
- High alpha-lactalbumin whey for sleep—10–20 g (as proteins+)

SUPPLEMENTS TO THE BRAIN DIET IN STRESS MANAGEMENT

- Rhodiola—180–300 mg (standardized to 3 percent rosavin—stress buffer)
- Ginkgo biloba—180 mg (GinkGold™—stress buffer)
- Ashwagandha—300 mg (standardized to 1.5 percent with ano-lides—stress buffer)
- High alpha-lactalbumin protein—10–20 g (e.g. proteins+—stress buffer and for sleep)

ATTENTION DEFICIT/HYPERACTIVITY DISORDER (ADHD)

As its name suggests, ADHD is characterized by a persistent pattern of inattention, hyperactivity, and/or impulsivity that impairs social, academic, or occupational functioning. Although best known in children, a growing number of adults are being diagnosed with ADHD. Symptoms usually manifest as disorganization, poor grades, poor productivity, mood swings, cognitive difficulties, temper flares, unusual sleeping patterns, impatience, and frequent interruption of others.

Obviously, when children and adults display such behaviors, appropriate human relationships can easily break down, and self-esteem suffers. Effective treatment is so critically important in ADHD because the long-term consequences can be catastrophic. In a follow-up study involving young boys who were diagnosed with ADHD at age seven, almost 60 percent at age twenty-two had problems with social adjustment: higher risks of antisocial behaviors, criminal records, alcohol abuse, reading difficulties, and low educational levels were noted. The standard medications for ADHD include stimulant- or amphetamine-like medications, most notably methylphenidate (Ritalin®). Scientists are continuing to work on the effectiveness of medications to treat ADHD.

The critics of medications for ADHD include celebrity types and others who are not involved in the direct care of ADHD patients. I have seen firsthand that these medications, and those for other psychiatric conditions, allow those with broken brains to function in life. No, the medications are not perfect, and they do come with side effects; however, they can make all the difference in the world to those who suffer from ADHD. I find it upsetting that doctors, parents, and children are made to feel bad about taking medications. Doctors themselves would prefer alternatives. A study in the *Journal of Managed Care Pharmacy* (2003) showed that the majority of prescribing doctors would prefer a non-controlled medication without evidence of abuse. However, stimulant medications do work, and 92 percent of those same physicians found them to be effective in treating ADHD. Consider that 75 percent of those who take the ADHD medications report improvement of symptoms, and for those parents, children, and teachers that is not a bad thing. Maybe the medication has allowed a young teen to go on to become a lawyer, or an adult to get the promotion she deserves. The focus should be on how we can make the current standard of care even better. The emerging research shows that nutritional interventions warrant serious consideration as part of the treatment plan in ADHD.

RESEARCH NOTES
- As previously discussed, the majority of research, including more recent and better-designed studies, have shown that there is a relationship between food additives and ADHD. Remove them. See the additive list at the Food and Behavior Research Web site, at www.fabresearch.org
- Children with ADHD respond to the glucose tolerance test in an abnormal way. The children present with a glucose "curve" that reflects hypoglycemia (low blood sugar), which fires up the sympathetic (stress) branch of the nervous system. Therefore, a short time after ingestion, large amounts of sugar cause a massive dive in blood glucose, which in turn stimulates stress hormone release. While ADHD patients appear to tolerate moderate levels of sugar, they may run in to trouble when they go beyond the average—which is already an incredible 40 to 50 teaspoons of sugar per day on average in North American children!
- In ADHD the emphasis should be on higher lean protein sources and lower amounts of non-fiber-containing carbohydrates. In other

words, increase the fish, lean poultry, and lean meat intake—and pass on the white bread, pasta, and cereals containing free toys.

- Vitamin B3 (niacin) may be helpful in ADHD.
- Vitamin B6 (pyridoxine) may be helpful in ADHD.
- Thiamine may be helpful in ADHD.
- Magnesium has been found to be low in ADHD.
- Zinc may be low in ADHD (strong evidence here).
- Calcium may be low in ADHD.
- Deficiency of essential fatty acids, particularly omega-3 fatty acids, seems to characterize ADHD. In 2003, Scottish researchers showed that children with ADHD break down omega-3 fatty acids more readily than healthy controls. The study, published in the journal *Nutritional Neuroscience*, used a noninvasive breath test to capture the oxidative damage to omega-3 fatty acids. The breath test may be valuable in determining the extent of oxidative stress-induced omega-3 damage in many brain disorders. I am told that test, by Pan Diagnostics, will be available in North America soon.
- Oxidative stress appears to be an issue in ADHD.
- Supplementation with omega-3 fatty acids and gamma-linolenic acid appears to benefit ADHD. However, the studies that used only DHA have not panned out well. Some EPA from fish oil appears to be required for therapeutic effect.
- While I am not suggesting it be used as a treatment, a number of studies show that caffeine is helpful in lowering ADHD. The point is that coffee or tea, at least in adults, may not have to be avoided—and the antioxidants within these beverages may actually be helpful.

SUPPLEMENTS TO THE BRAIN DIET IN ADHD

- Essential fatty acids—research in children aged 5–12 has used 500 mg EPA, 200 mg DHA, 60 mg GLA. Adults may consider higher amounts (double) of all the essential fatty acids. Adult ADHD may require 1000 mg to 2000 mg of EPA. Flax oil may not be converted well into EPA and DHA in the liver of ADHD patients according to Canadian research. Prioritize fish oil, e.g., o3mega+ think™.
- Zinc sulfate—providing at least 15 mg and up to 45 mg of elemental (actual) zinc. These levels were used in studies with children approximately 10 years old.
- Ginkgo biloba and American ginseng—400 mg of American ginseng and 100 mg of ginkgo. Average age in study was ten years old.
- Magnesium citrate—100 mg children, 300 mg adults.

AUTISM AND RELATED DISORDERS

Autism is a neurological condition of early childhood; it manifests as impairment in social interactions and communication. There are also signs of repetitive and stereotyped patterns of behavior. The cause of autism remains unknown. However, genetics do appear to play a role in many cases. Other conditions related to autism, the so-called pervasive developmental disorders, include Rett's disorder (more movement difficulties) and Asperger's disorder (normal language and cognitive development).

Researchers are now beginning to direct considerable attention to autism as the rates have been rising dramatically over the last decade. Some of the statistics are alarming, although a greater overall awareness of the condition may be driving the diagnoses. In the United States, the overall rates increased from 18 percent to 26 percent in recent years. California seems to have an inordinate number of new cases of autism: the state saw a 97 percent increase in autism between the late 1990s and 2002 and a 31 percent increase from 2001 to 2002 alone. In Canada, the Ministry of Education of Quebec noted a 63 percent increase in autism or related disorders from 2001 to 2003. Similar elevations in autism rates have been noted in regions of the U.K. and the Middle East, and a significant rise in Japan has recently been reported.

Fingers have been pointed at infant vaccines, but there is no clear indication that any relationship exists. Still, we need to continue to look at the environment to determine why rates are increasing so much. It is unlikely that these sharp global rises are purely related to awareness, or a "trendy diagnosis," as inappropriately suggested in New Scientist (August 13–19, 2005). It is much more likely that something in our environment is pushing the increase in genetically susceptible individuals.

One environmental factor that has certainly increased over the last decade is the use of computers, the construction of cell phone towers, and the keeping of cell phones in the vicinity of pregnant women. I am not alone in observing this possible connection. Dr. Robert Kane published his thesis on the connection between enhanced electromagnetic frequency radiation (EMF) and the increase in autism. His research, published in Medical Hypotheses (2004), is an urgent call to investigate any possible connection between EMF exposure and autism.

One recent piece of research found that, like most brain conditions, inflammation is part of the process in autism. At this point it is unclear if inflammation is the cause or the consequence of the condition, but in any case, an anti-inflammatory diet is in order. As previously mentioned, there are also disturbances in the intestinal bacteria, and probiotics might have a place in treatment. As with ADHD, a number of studies have shown that autistic patients are under increased oxidative stress and that levels of omega-3 fatty acids are diminished. High-quality nutrition is critical in autism because the behavioral problems and repetitive behaviors can set the stage for eating only a few foods—and obviously, without a varied diet the loss of key brain nutrients can occur.

NUTRITIONAL CONSIDERATIONS
- Low intakes of vitamins A, B1 (thiamine), B3 (niacin), B5 (pantothenic acid), B6, and B12 have been noted in autism.
- Biotin levels may be low.
- Selenium intake is subpar.
- Zinc intake is low.
- Magnesium intake is low.
- Essential fatty acids, particularly omega-3 fatty acids, have been shown to be low in autism.

SUPPLEMENTS TO THE BRAIN DIET IN AUTISM
- Essential fatty acids—500 mg EPA and 300 mg DHA; clinical trials are under way to investigate fish oils
- Magnesium—dose to be set by body weight
- Vitamin C—dose to be set by body weight
- Folic acid—dose to be set by body weight
- Vitamin B12—dose to be set by body weight
- Probiotics—30 billion colony forming units of *Lactobacillus* GG (Culturelle), 5 billion cfu of *Lactobacillus plantarum* 299V, 1 billion cfu of Life Start (Natren), 4 mg of *Bifidobacterium infantis* 35624 (Align™)

ALZHEIMER'S DISEASE AND DEMENTIA

Dementia is characterized by multiple cognitive deficits such as impaired memory, judgment, learning, reasoning, orientation, and communication. There are many causes of dementia, many of them related to brain

disease or traumatic injury. Alzheimer's disease is a progressive neurological condition involving the buildup of amyloid plaque just outside brain
cells and abnormal protein structures inside the nerve cells called neu-
rofibrillary tangles. Alzheimer's patients lose brain cells and the small
gaps between nerve cells (synapses) are also wiped out, a situation that
obviously impairs normal communication between cells.

Alzheimer's disease (AD) accounts for about 70 percent of all demen-
tia-related conditions. For now, the lifetime risk of AD is 19 percent for
women and 10 percent for men over age sixty-five. The prevalence of AD
is expected to at least quadruple in the next forty years, and given the
new connections between AD and obesity, the numbers might end up
being much higher.

Make no mistake about it, Alzheimer's disease is an absolutely heart-
wrenching condition, particularly for loved ones who progressively lose
their spouse or family member. AD patients often experience profound
personality changes and ultimately lose the ability to take care of themselves. The AD wheels are set in motion many years before the dramatic
behavioral and mental changes take place. It is now known that depression and low-level chronic inflammation may increase the risk of later
AD. As with most brain-related conditions, oxidative stress/damage plays
a significant role in AD.

A diet top-heavy in acidic foods (too much animal protein) may be
the reason why there is diminished bone-mineral density and increased
aluminum uptake in Alzheimer's disease. Alkaline fruits and vegetables
contain potassium and magnesium, which may act as a "buffer" to prevent
aluminum absorption. While there are conflicting reports on the overall
impact of aluminum on the pathology of AD, one thing is pretty clear at
this point: patients with AD absorb significantly more aluminum than
healthy controls, and that is never a good thing. It is also certain that aluminum promotes inflammation and oxidative stress. While much has
been made of aluminum in water, deodorants, and pots and pans, it
appears that processed foods are a far more significant source (more than
ten times more) of aluminum for North Americans. Aluminum can occur
naturally in food and water, but it is greatly amplified in the form of baking powder, anticaking agents, emulsifiers, thickeners, leaveners, and sta-
bilizers. A study in the journal *Age and Aging* (1999) showed a
significantly higher risk of AD in consumers of pancakes, waffles, biscuits,

muffins, cornbread, and corn tortillas. In a 2005 study in *Food Additives and Contaminants* it was shown that a serving of restaurant pancakes provides a whopping 182 mg of aluminum. More research is needed in this area, but for now awareness of the aluminum in diet is important.

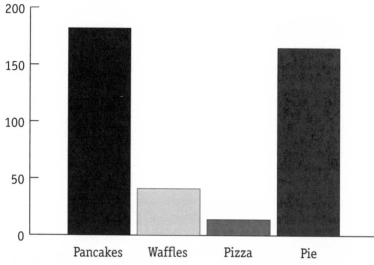

Aluminum content in milligrams per serving: restaurant pancakes, frozen waffles, frozen pizza, and frozen raspberry pie. (Saiyed, et al. *Food Additives and Contaminants*, 2005; 22:234–44)

NUTRITIONAL CONSIDERATIONS

- The diet that appears to afford the greatest protection against cognitive decline involves fibrous carbohydrates, whole grain cereals, nuts, red wine, fruits and vegetables, and marine-based fats.

- When Japanese people move to the United States and adopt a more Western diet and lifestyle, their risk of dementia rises dramatically. One study showed that Japanese-American men living in the United States have a two and a half times higher risk of Alzheimer's disease versus matched controls in Japan.

- Early studies showed that higher total fat intake increases the risk of AD. As research becomes more sophisticated, it appears that animal fat is the culprit.

- Individuals who develop AD tend to consume greater overall calories and less fruits and vegetables in the years before onset.

- The omega-6 fatty acid linoleic acid (found in corn, soybean, safflower, and sunflower oils) is associated with cognitive impairment.

- Monounsaturated fats, found in nuts and olive oil, reduce the risk of cognitive decline.
- Fish and marine-based omega-3 are associated with a reduced risk of cognitive decline and AD.
- Higher cholesterol increases the risk of AD.
- Low levels of vitamins B6 and B12, thiamine, riboflavin, and folic acid have been associated with cognitive decline.
- Low levels of vitamin C are associated with worse memory and cognitive performance in older people.
- Low intake of dietary antioxidants is associated with increased risk of cognitive decline. Vitamins C and E from dietary sources are valuable in protecting against dementia, while isolated supplements appear to offer little to no protection. A combination of supplemental antioxidants has been associated with a reduced risk of AD, according to research in the *Archives of Neurology* (2004). The message is clear: Antioxidants work together, so do not expect taking vitamin E alone or vitamin C alone to do much for you.

SUPPLEMENTS TO THE BRAIN DIET IN COGNITIVE DECLINE

- Carnosine and Taurine—1000 mg and 400 mg respectively daily (as Life Extension™ Super Carnosine)
- Acetyl-L-carnitine and alpha-lipoic acid—as Juvenon™, 2 capsules daily
- EPA/DHA—1000 mg daily (as o3mega+think™)
- Phosphatidylsesine—300 mg daily
- Ginkgo biloba—240 mg daily (as Ginkgold™)
- DHEA—10–25 mg—see your doctor
- Huperzine A (Hup A)—400 mcg daily; clinical trials in China have demonstrated efficacy; U.S. studies are under way

BED-WETTING—ENURESIS

Bed-wetting is an extremely distressing condition, particularly when it occurs beyond the age of seven. The negative psychological impact on children and their families has been well described in the scientific literature. Although bed-wetting can be brought on in children after traumatic events, cases of primary nocturnal enuresis (night wetting with no extended dry period) is now documented as an organic brain condition. Children with primary bed-wetting have been shown to have a lack of inhibition in the brain area which initiates urination. Bed-wetting does spontaneously resolve for most young children and adolescents over the years, and this appears to reflect a slower maturation of some brain areas.

In addition, children with primary bed-wetting have elevations in inflammatory chemicals called prostaglandins and nitric oxide. These chemicals cause children with bed-wetting to dump off higher amounts of sodium and magnesium into urine, which in turn increases the overall volume and nocturnal voiding. Medications that inhibit the prostaglandins and nitric oxide are helpful in children with bed-wetting, but they don't address the brain area which initiates urination. This is where omega-3 fatty acids, and EPA in particular, might play a significant role.

The ability of EPA to inhibit prostaglandins and nitric oxide in the kidneys is well documented, both experimentally in animals and in humans as well. Therefore, EPA may prevent excessive nocturnal urinary volume and prevent voiding. The added bonus is that omega-3 fatty acids, at least experimentally, can prevent the delay in normal inhibition of different areas in the brain.

Omega-3 deficiency can cause a delay in other inhibitory centers in the vicinity of the brain's urination center. The rates of bed-wetting in children are much higher in the United States, United Kingdom, Turkey, and Australia versus Malaysia, Korea, and Taiwan. It may not surprise you that the latter three countries consume at least more than double the fish and seafood per person each year. Nutrition, in the form of omega-3 fatty acids, may influence the genetics of bed-wetting.

In 2005, Dr. Francois Lesperance of the University of Montreal and I published our rationale for the study of omega-3 fatty acids and bed-wetting in the journal *Medical Hypotheses*. There is every reason to suspect that omega-3 fatty acids may be of real value to those children who need more than the current treatment options.

From a behavioral perspective, it has been noted that most children with bed-wetting do not drink much in the earlier part of the day, and consume more fluids after 5:00 p.m. It makes no sense to restrict fluid at night with this pattern in place because children can become dangerously dehydrated. Expert Dr. Mark Jalkut and colleagues from UCLA suggest that children drink 40 percent of their fluids before noon, 40 percent before 4:30 p.m., and only 20 percent in the evening. Beverages containing caffeine are off limits.

Nutritional Considerations

- Bed-wetting may be a signal that omega-3 fatty acids are in deficiency. There is a significant overlap between childhood disorders
  such as ADHD (where omega-3 fatty acids have been helpful) and
  primary bed-wetting.

- Food sensitivities may play a role in bed-wetting, which is not all
  that surprising given the new findings of low-level inflammation
  induced by food intolerances. The immune chemicals (cytokines)
  induced by food intolerances can promote the production of the
  prostaglandins and nitric oxide involved in bed-wetting. In a study
  in *Clinical Pediatrics* (1992), researchers from the Hospital for Sick
  Children in London showed that removal of certain foods and food
  chemicals improved bed-wetting in children an average of seven
  years of age. Reintroduction of one or more foods caused a relapse
  in bed-wetting. Chocolate, oranges, cow's milk, benzoic acid, and
  tartrazine (food additives) were the main culprits.

Supplements to the Brain Diet in Enuresis (Bed-Wetting)

- EPA omega-3—500–1000 mg (as o3mega+joy™ or
  o3mega+think™)
- Zinc—15 g
- Magnesium—100 mg

CHRONIC FATIGUE SYNDROME/FIBROMYALGIA

Chronic fatigue syndrome (CFS) is a relatively common disorder, particularly in women, affecting 522 women and 291 men per 100,000. There
are many symptoms of CFS, including headache, joint pain, cognitive
disturbances, gastrointestinal (GI) concerns, visual disturbances, dizziness, and others. Involvement of the brain and central nervous system in
CFS is a legitimate feature of the illness. Abnormalities on MRI and
other brain-imaging tests have been documented in a growing number of
studies. Problems with blood flow to the brain, inner-ear functioning, and
gait (walking) have all been documented. In addition, there is no shortage of research showing that CFS patients have elevations in those
immune chemicals (cytokines) that can disturb mood, cognition, and
promote low-level inflammation and fatigue.

Fibromyalgia (FM) is a commonly diagnosed rheumatic condition
that affects more women than men. The prevalence of FM is approximately 3,400 women and 500 men per 100,000. In women, those numbers rival cardiovascular disease and arthritis. FM is characterized by

widespread pain, fatigue, GI complaints, insomnia, cognitive difficulties, and many other symptoms. The overlap between CFS and FM symptoms is very, very high, to the point that some experts consider them to be the same illnesses. There are also significant overlaps between CFS/FM and migraine headaches, irritable bowel syndrome, and anxiety/depressive disorders. The depressive symptoms most often appear after the illness onset, and that should be expected given the severe impact of the illness on the lives of those who were normally high-functioning individuals. Patients with CFS/FM frequently use dietary modifications (exclusion of some foods, inclusion of others) and 70 percent report that a healthy diet is important in managing the illness.

NUTRITIONAL CONSIDERATIONS

- At least four published studies have suggested that a vegetarian or vegan (no dairy or eggs) diet can improve the symptoms of FM. Decreased pain and joint stiffness, improved sleep quality, physical performance, mental health, and overall well-being have all been noted.

- Improvements in FM symptoms have been associated with increased antioxidant status and improved intestinal bacterial profile. Remember that both CFS and FM are well documented to have small intestinal bacterial overgrowth (SIBO).

- The vegetarian/vegan studies may have had improvements because they included liberal consumption of fruits, vegetables, nuts, seeds, sprouts, and dark pigmented berries such as cranberry, blueberry, and blackcurrant.

- Despite the benefits of vegan/vegetarian diets, most FM patients returned to old eating habits over time when the studies concluded. The message is that moderate changes to the diet may be more likely to lead to higher compliance. Elevation in the intake of a variety of fruits and vegetables and a reduction in the intake of inflammatory animal fat is central to the Brain Diet.

- We have talked about advanced glycation endproducts (AGE) in this book and the importance of keeping dietary AGE to minimal levels. FM patients have been shown to have elevated AGE production in the body. Additional dietary AGE burden is obviously not a good thing.

- Fish oil has been shown to improve symptoms in patients with both CFS and FM.

- Removal of monosodium glutamate (MSG) and aspartame was shown to dramatically improve symptoms of FM, and worsen them upon challenge with these same additives. The study, published in the *Annals of Pharmacotherapy* (2001), suggests that these and other chemicals are gaining rapid access to the nervous system via a porous blood-brain barrier.

- Again, as with many brain-related conditions, it is worth investigating food intolerances in CFS and FM. A number of university-based studies have shown that certain foods appear to provoke symptoms in CFS and FM. For more on these studies, see *Hope and Help for Chronic Fatigue Syndrome and Fibromyalgia* by Dr. Alison Bested (Cumberland House, 2006).

- Make sure your doctor eliminates celiac disease as a diagnosis. Celiac disease (severe intolerance to a wheat protein) is underdiagnosed and may actually present without GI symptoms and with only brain-related symptoms.

- Magnesium levels may be low in CFS/FM.

- Omega-3 fatty acids may be low in CFS/FM; EPA has been shown to be helpful.

- Thiamine (vitamin B1), folic acid, vitamin B12, and zinc may be low in CFS/FM.

- Co-enzyme Q10 may be low. Supplementation with ginkgo and CoQ10 in FM has been shown to be helpful.

SUPPLEMENTS TO THE BRAIN DIET IN CFS/FM

- EPA—1000–2000mg (as o3mega+joy™)
- Acetyl-L-carnitine and alpha-lipoic acid—2 capsules Juvenon™ daily
- NADH—10 mg daily (as Enada™)
- Magnesium citrate—500 mg daily
- Co-enzyme Q10—100 mg daily
- Ginkgo biloba—180–240 mg daily (as Ginkgold™)
- 5HTP—300 mg daily (for FM pain and insomnia)

IRRITABLE BOWEL SYNDROME

Irritable bowel syndrome (IBS) is the most common disorder of the GI tract. Symptoms of IBS include abdominal discomfort/pain, constipation and/or alternating diarrhea, and bloating and abdominal distention for extended periods. It is estimated that about one quarter of North Americans will experience IBS in the course of a lifetime. For many, the onset follows a gastrointestinal infection. IBS leads to an estimated 3.5 million visits to physicians each year—with many, many more never visiting a health-care provider for treatment. IBS has significant overlap with psychiatric conditions, most notably anxiety and depression. IBS is considered in the Brain Diet because there are now signs of dysfunction within the "brain" that resides in the gut. The small intestinal bacterial overgrowth, the alterations in beneficial bacterial numbers, and the signs of chronic low-level inflammation in IBS point to a benefit from the Brain Diet.

NUTRITIONAL CONSIDERATIONS

- Dietary fiber as a supplement or dietary intake could go either way. Some studies suggest benefits, others show a worsening of symptoms. Increasing fiber in the form of fruits and vegetables should be a priority, then try more digestible cereal-based fiber (e.g., cooked oatmeal), then "hard" insoluble wheat-based fiber (e.g., wheat bran cereals). Experimentation with fiber is worthwhile.

- Volatile oils from plants, particularly peppermint oil, can help to normalize the rhythmic movements of the intestinal tract.

- Many cases of IBS may in fact be lactose intolerance. Removal of dairy and other sources of lactose are worth investigating.

- Limitation of simple dietary sugars, including fructose, may improve symptoms. With small intestinal bacterial overgrowth (SIBO) common to IBS, such simple carbohydrates might enter the colon undigested and cause multiple symptoms.

- Anti-inflammatory foods components, turmeric in particular, has been shown to be of benefit.

- Food components that promote the growth of beneficial bacteria, such as artichoke, may be of benefit.

SUPPLEMENTATION TO THE BRAIN DIET IN IBS

- Probiotics—First choice is 1–2 capsules (4–8 mg) *Bifidobacterium infantis* 35624 (Align™). If no improvement, try alternating *Lactobacillus* GG (Culturelle) and *Lactobacillus plantarum* 299V—1 capsule each daily.

- Enteric-coated peppermint oil—0.2ml three times a day between meals (as Pepogest™)

- Turmeric extract—300 mg two to three times with a meal

- Artichoke extract—300 mg two to three times with a meal

- Melatonin—3 mg improves abdominal and rectal pain

MIGRAINE HEADACHES

Migraine headaches are characterized by throbbing pain that typically affects only one side of the head. Onset is sudden, and while the precise mechanisms are not fully defined, there is constriction and then dilation of the blood vessels surrounding the brain, which irritates nerves and causes explosive pain. Migraines can occur with an uncomfortable warning called an aura, or there may be no feeling in advance. Either way, the end result is extreme pain often accompanied by nausea and other bodily symptoms. Migraine is associated with an increased risk of anxiety (phobias and panic attacks) and depression. My colleague Dr. Alison Bested and I found that half of a large population of chronic fatigue syndrome patients had migraine headaches before CFS onset.

Abnormal levels of the neurochmical serotonin may initiate the constriction of blood vessels. Since foods containing serotonin (banana, avocado, walnut, pineapple, kiwi) are among the foods that might trigger migraines, a look at the diet for sensitivities is worthwhile. Patients with migraine headaches have been shown to have intestinal permeability— chemicals getting through the gut barrier that should not be. In addition, it is likely that the perimeter fence around the brain, the blood-brain barrier, is also more porous. This contributes to the sensitivity to various foods and food additives.

Nutritional Considerations

- Caffeine withdrawal may be a trigger, and yet because it constricts blood vessels, it may help with an acute attack. Those with migraines should exercise caution with caffeine.
- Magnesium deficiency may be involved in migraine.
- Vitamin B12 deficiency may be involved.
- Omega-3 fatty acids and GLA from borage oil may be helpful.
- Aspartame and monosodium glutamate (MSG) may cause migraines in certain individuals. Nitrites in preserved meats may also be a culprit; restriction may be helpful.
- Avoidance of serotonin-containing foods may be worth trying.
- Ginger inhibits a specific serotonin receptor, the 5HT3 receptor. Scientists have shown that medications that block this receptor are valuable in the treatment of migraine. Although ginger has not yet been investigated in modern clinical trials, it does have a long history of use in India as a migraine treatment.

- Limitation of simple carbohydrates and sugars is prudent. Many patients with migraine report onset when blood sugar is low. Simple sugars, sweets, soft drinks, etc., spike sugar—but it is short-lived, and a large drop-off can follow.
- Dysfunction of the energy packs of the cells (mitochondria) may be involved in migraine headaches. Preliminary research suggests that co-enzyme Q10 and vitamin B12 are effective.

SUPPLEMENTS TO THE BRAIN DIET IN MIGRAINE

- Magnesium citrate—300 mg daily
- EPA—1000 mg daily (as o3mega+joy™)
- Riboflavin (vitamin B2)—400 mg daily
- 5-HTP—200–300 mg daily
- Feverfew herb—minimum 0.25 mg of parthenolide daily
- Butterbur herb—minimum 75 mg extract containing at least 15 percent petasins
- Ginger syrup—2 teaspoons (as Ginger Wonder™)
- Co-enzyme Q10—150 mg daily

MULTIPLE SCLEROSIS

Multiple sclerosis (MS) is a chronic autoimmune condition that is most likely triggered by environmental factors in those who may be genetically susceptible. In MS there is an attack on the nerve cells by the body's own immune system. Specifically, the immune cells go after the myelin sheath, a fatty insulator that surrounds nerve fibers. With enough damage, communication within and between nerve cells is slowed and ultimately blocked. Chronic inflammation is a hallmark of MS. The symptoms of MS include difficulty in walking, balance and coordination problems, cognitive dysfunction, visual disturbances, headaches, numbness, and pain.

A number of triggers have been proposed, including viruses and other microbial agents. Much has been made of latitude regarding MS. There are much higher rates in the northern United States and northern Europe versus southern regions of the United States and the European continent. This might seem to suggest a weather/climate connection. However, much like seasonal affective disorder, it does not always hold true. For example, the Inuit and native populations of northern polar regions and the Japanese at higher latitudes have extremely low rates of MS and seasonal affective disorder. I think you can guess at least one dietary item that the Japanese and the native/Inuit populations have in common—yes, it is fish and other marine foods.

NUTRITIONAL CONSIDERATIONS

- The nations with low rates of MS maintain a diet high in omega-3 fatty acids and close to traditional diets low in animal fat. Even within nations, there are significant dietary differences associated with MS risk. For example, the diets of those living in the coastal regions of Norway were found to be much higher in fish and seafood, while in the inland regions, where rates of MS were eight times higher, residents consumed much greater amounts of dairy and animal fat.

- According to the research of physician Roy Swank, animal fat is a significant culprit in MS. In his long-term follow-up study published in *Nutrition* (2003), Dr. Swank and colleague Dr. James Goodwin showed that 20 percent of those in an animal fat–restricted diet had little or no progression of the illness at all. They also noted that overall, if saturated fat was kept very low, MS patients had excellent long-term survival and mobility to advanced age. Note that supplementation of omega-3 fatty acid was advised along with the saturated fat restriction.

- Separate investigators have found that milk, animal fat, smoked meat, and white potato are dietary factors associated with an increased risk of MS.

- Omega-3 EPA and DHA levels have been found to be low in MS.

- Fish and vegetable intake have been associated with a decreased risk.

- Small studies suggest benefit from omega-3 fish oil and GLA.

- Low levels of B12 have been noted in MS.

- Calcium and magnesium supplementation may be of benefit.

- Although often recommended, there is no evidence that a gluten-free diet should be adhered to. While it is absolutely worth investigating food intolerances in MS, it should be noted that a gluten-free diet actually worsened the condition in the animal model of MS.

- Vegetables containing the phytochemical luteolin may be extremely valuable in MS. New experimental research shows that luteolin prevents myelin breakdown and improves symptoms in the animal model of MS. Luteolin is found in high amounts in artichokes, celery, and parsley.

- The latitude connection with MS may be related to a protective role of vitamin D. Indeed MS patients have been noted to have low levels of vitamin D. Higher dietary and supplemental vitamin D was associated with a 33 to 40 percent reduction in MS risk among more than ninety thousand women followed for twenty years.

SUPPLEMENTS TO THE BRAIN DIET IN MULTIPLE SCLEROSIS

- EPA—1000 mg to 2000 mg daily (as o3mega+joy™)
- Calcium citrate—1000 mg daily
- Magnesium citrate—300 mg daily
- Gamma-linolenic acid—500 mg daily (from borage oil or evening primrose oil)
- Vitamin B12—10–30 mg (in the form of methylcobalamin)
- Alpha-lipoic acid and acetyl-L-carnitine—2 capsules daily (as Juvenon™)

INSOMNIA

We have previously discussed the importance of quality sleep in maintaining not only mental sharpness but also a healthy body weight. Surveys of North Americans indicate that half of all adults report sleep difficulties, and of them, 36 percent report that they have been dealing with sleep problems for more than one year. Sadly, only 9 percent of patients with sleep difficulties discuss the issue with their primary physician. In addition to the cognitive difficulties and possible long-term weight gain, those with insomnia have a twenty times higher risk of developing depression. Also, having insomnia within a brain-related condition, both neurological and psychiatric, usually worsens the outcome. Clearly, sleep is life-giving, and it is critical for mental performance. Dietary measures may be helpful in the induction and the maintenance of sleep.

NUTRITIONAL CONSIDERATION

- Caffeine in food and beverages may interfere with sleep. Individual variations are apparent; some can consume more caffeine than others without ill effects on sleep. However, the influence of caffeine in cases of insomnia and anxiety is a reality that is often overlooked. Large-scale research shows that, incredibly, those taking sleeping and anxiety medications do not differ in caffeine intake compared to healthy controls. One would think that caffeine limitation would be found in the insomnia group as they should be making efforts to limit caffeine.

- Food restriction is known to interfere with sleep onset and quality. That said, the way to induce sleep is not via a heavy late-evening or nighttime meal. A small carbohydrate snack might be just enough, whole grain toast, or a small bowl of cereal may boost sleep-inducing brain serotonin levels.

- A warm glass of milk was traditionally recommended for sleep, and now nutritional scientists have identified the sleep-inducing protein from milk and shown it to be effective. The milk protein alpha-lactalbumin (ALA) is particularly rich in tryptophan, the amino acid required for the manufacture of serotonin in the brain. Tryptophan has restricted access to the brain because other large amino acids in the blood compete for uptake into the brain. However, if you can elevate the blood tryptophan to large neutral amino acids (Try:LNAA) ratio by 40 or 50 percent, you can increase serotonin in the brain. A recent study in the *American Journal of Clinical Nutrition* (2005) showed that ALA increased the blood Try:LNAA ratio by a whopping 130 percent in healthy adults. Those same adults taking ALA in the evening reported improved morning alertness and cognitive function the following day. The researchers suggested the effects were due to improved sleep via higher brain serotonin. These results support earlier animal studies showing a sleep-inducing effect of ALA, and human research showing a stress-buffering effect.

- Magnesium deficiency may accompany insomnia.

- Thiamine (vitamin B1) may assist sleep quality.

- Vitamin B12 may assist sleep quality.

- Alcohol may be sedating, but it interferes with sleep quality.

Supplements to the Brain Diet in Insomnia

- High alpha-lactalbumin whey protein—20–40 g
- Melatonin—0.5 to 6 mg (start low and work up slowly)
- Vitamin B12—500 mcg (as methylcobalamin)
- Magnesium citrate—300 mg
- 5-HTP—100–300 mg (evening use; do not take with alpha-lactalbumin, may cause too much serotonin production and accumulation)
- Valerian—200–400 mg at bedtime (standardized extract)
- Passion flower—200 mg at bedtime (standardized extract)

PARKINSON'S DISEASE

Parkinson's disease (PD) is a degenerative disorder of the central nervous system. There are close to one million North Americans with PD, with an increasing frequency of individuals under sixty being diagnosed with this progressive condition. The symptoms of the illness are a result of selective degeneration of nerve cells in the area of the brain called the substantia nigra. Without proper production and usage of the neurotransmitter dopamine, the PD patient experiences tremors at rest, slow movements, rigidity, and difficulty with walking and maintaining posture.

NUTRITIONAL CONSIDERATIONS

- Increased intake of animal fat is associated with increased risk of PD.
- Increased risk of PD with increased iron intake (this may also implicate red meat as a source of iron and animal fat).
- Increased risk of PD with higher intake of cholesterol (again, red meat is a source of animal fat, iron, and cholesterol).
- Higher overall calorie intake earlier in life increases PD risk.
- Nuts have been noted as protective.
- Plums (very high antioxidant fruit) have been shown to be associated with a reduced risk of PD.
- Omega-3 fatty acids (in the form of cod liver oil) have been noted to be protective when consumed during early life.
- High does of riboflavin (vitamin B2) and elimination of dietary red meat has been shown to promote the recovery of motor functions in PD patients.
- Taurine is low in PD patients.
- Coffee consumption is protective against PD.
- Polyunsaturated fats are protective against PD.
- Creatine may be helpful in PD.
- Dysfunction of the energy packets of the cells (mitochondria) and oxidative stress appear to play a large role in PD. A host of studies using the animal model of PD show that antioxidants and agents that support mitochondrial function are protective. Examples include ginkgo, acetyl-L-carnitine and co-enzyme Q10. Co-Q10 has been shown to be helpful in new human trials with PD patients.

SUPPLEMENTS TO THE BRAIN DIET IN PARKINSON'S DISEASE

- Acetyl-L-carnitine and alpha-lipoic acid—2 to 4 capsules daily (Juvenon™)
- Co-enzyme Q10—500–1000 mg daily
- NADH—10–30 mg daily (Enada™)
- Taurine—1000 mg daily

- EPA—1000 mg daily (o3mega+joy™)
- Zinc sulfate—30 mg daily

SCHIZOPHRENIA

Schizophrenia is a brain condition characterized by delusions, hallucinations, and disorganized speech and behavior. Patients with schizophrenia often withdraw socially; they may have so-called negative symptoms where there is little or no emotional expression (flat affect). Those with schizophrenia may adopt a very unhealthy lifestyle, particularly when the disease progresses. There is no shortage of research showing that schizophrenia is indeed a very physical condition of the brain. There are countless studies showing alterations in brain structures, nerve cell chemicals, and physiology. Genetics appears to account for about 30 percent of the illness, and given that it does not occur in equal geographic distribution, all arrows point to environmental factors—one of which may be nutritional.

Nutritional Considerations

- Those with schizophrenia eat a diet higher in fat and low in fiber.
- High consumption of sugar and saturated fat has been associated with worse outcomes over the long term.
- High intake of meat and dairy has been associated with worse outcome in schizophrenia.
- Rates of schizophrenia are lower, and outcome is better, in Asian nations where fish and seafood consumption is typically higher, and sugar consumption is typically lower than that in the West.
- Many studies have documented increased oxidative stress in schizophrenia. The oxidative stress quickly uses up antioxidant vitamins (e.g., vitamin C) which may be the reason for low blood levels.
- Blood sugar abnormalities and insulin resistance also appear to be related to the condition.
- Low levels of eicosapentaenoic acid (EPA) omega-3 are associated with more severe symptoms.
- Four out of five studies using EPA have shown at least some benefit in symptoms.
- Nutrients that regulate essential fatty acid metabolism, including zinc, selenium, and vitamin B6 may be helpful in schizophrenia.

SUPPLEMENTS TO THE BRAIN DIET IN SCHIZOPHRENIA

- EPA—2000–3000 mg daily (as o3mega+joy™)
- Vitamin C—1000 mg daily
- Zinc—15 mg daily

Closing Remarks

The human diet must provide both fuel and protection for our delicate nerve cells, the very cells that drive our thoughts, actions, beliefs, emotions, and desires. These same cells can sabotage our lives if not fully supported. The fallout of unsupported nerve cells can be dramatic. Remember that the brain and nerve cells produce violence, aggression, depression, anxiety, impulsivity, and other (for the most part) undesirable emotions and behaviors. In early life, the brain and nerve cells, if not properly developed, can rob our children of normal human emotional and intellectual growth and normal human relationships. Later in life, unprotected and nutritionally unsupported brain and nerve cells leave us a mere shell of our former selves, impairing our memory and mobility.

From the moment of conception through the best of the golden years, we must support the conductor of the orchestra known as the human body. The stakes are very high. A healthy brain, functioning in top gear, is an important prerequisite to maximizing our quality of life. Think of what we do in our lives for our children and our own future. We try to better our lot in life and do the most for our children—the best schools, the best tutors, after-school activities, sporting events, music, career development, and entertainment to name just a few. We always want "the best" for our kids. The time to prioritize nutritional health as a means of maximizing the full potential of our children is now. There are urgent nutritional voids that must be filled in, and other areas such as excess sugar, saturated and trans fats, and excess calories in general that must be limited—their brain and their future depend on it, particularly in today's increasingly competitive world.

As adults, we push ourselves in so many areas of our lives: we save, we invest, we buy insurance, and we try to make choices that are for the good of today, and for the good of our future. Given the emerging research on nutritional influences on brain-related conditions, we should also consider our dietary choices as an investment in our future. Adhering to the Brain Diet plan can help to maximize daily cognitive performance, maintain a healthy outlook, and enhance overall well-being.

A diet rich in colorful fruits and vegetables, oily fish, seafood, and whole grains can provide the fiber, antioxidants, and healthy fats that prevent inflammation and oxidative stress from taking its toll. We can also take advantage of beneficial bacteria to promote proper intestinal health and Brassica vegetables to promote detoxification. Research now indicates that nutrition can influence genetic expression—whether or not, or to what degree, an individual may experience a particular condition. These same dietary components that protect our brain cells may influence the delicate genetic material inside.

We should also make appropriate choices with regard to certain produce that may contain high levels of environmental chemicals and certain fish that may contain mercury or other contaminants. Maintaining a lean body will help to maximize brain function, and this is where mind-body medicine is invaluable. Often overlooked, the environmental context in which eating takes place can promote stress and drive inappropriate food choices. Using stress management will not only help to limit the production of brain-damaging immune and adrenal gland chemicals, it will help to limit overeating and/or making the wrong choices when it comes to brain-friendly foods.

Dietary supplements can make a valuable contribution to the Brain Diet in the promotion of brain health. Filling in the nutritional voids with food-based phytochemicals, fiber, omega-3 fatty acids, and a high-quality multivitamin/mineral formula should be prioritized. Specialty supplements should be reserved for use after the basic nutritional issues are taken care of. Supplements are never a substitute for making every effort to maximize your intake of brain-friendly foods. Supplements are also not a substitute for appropriate mental health or neurological care. Guidance from a health-care provider should be part of any supplement plan when it is directed at a brain-related condition.

We have taken many twists and turns through the pages of the Brain Diet, from gaping nutritional voids in our diet, the inflammation/oxidative stress connection, the obesity influence, environmental toxins, and the health of the gut. There are many areas of science that appear, at least on the surface, not to be connected at all. However, when you start to connect the scientific dots by drawing on research from a number of disciplines, amazing networks start to come together. It is like one of those 3D puzzle posters you stare at for a while and then the picture inside jumps out at you; in this case, the image is the human brain.

Remember, when you shop and prepare meals for yourself or your family, there are powerful choices to be made, choices that can influence the brain today, tomorrow, and well into the future.

Appendix: Resources

NUTRITION UPDATES

www.drlogan.com

BRAIN-RELATED MEDICAL CONDITIONS

National Institute of Mental Health (NIMH)
Public Information and Communications
Branch
6001 Executive Boulevard, Room 8184,
MSC 9663
Bethesda, MD 20892-9663
(301) 443-4513
(866) 615-6464 (toll-free)
(301) 443-8431 (TTY)
(866) 415-8051 (TTY toll-free)

National Institute of Neurological Disorders
P.O. Box 5801
Bethesda, MD 20824
(301) 496-5751
(800) 352-9424 (toll-free)
(301) 468-5981 (TTY)

Anxiety and Phobia Treatment Center at
White Plains Hospital
Davis Avenue at East Post Road
White Plains, NY 10601
(914) 681-1038
www.phobia-anxiety.org
Support groups and anxiety/stress
management courses

NUTRITIONALLY ORIENTED MEDICAL DOCTORS
AND NATUROPATHIC PHYSICIANS

American Holistic Medical Association
12101 Menaul Blvd., NE, Suite C
Albuquerque, NM 87112
(505) 292-7788
Fax: (505) 293-7582
http://www.holisticmedicine.org

The American Association of Naturopathic
Physicians
3201 New Mexico Avenue, NW
Suite 350
Washington, DC 20016
(202) 895-1392
(866) 538-2267 (toll-free)
Fax: (202) 274-1992
http://www.naturopathic.org

Canadian Association of Naturopathic Doctors
1255 Sheppard Ave. E., Toronto
Canada M2K1E2
(416) 496-8633
(800) 551-4381 (toll-free)
Fax: (416) 496-8634
http://www.naturopathicassoc.ca

MIND-BODY MEDICINE PROGRAMS AND
RESOURCES

Harvard Mind-Body Medical Institute
Programs
824 Boylston St.
Chestnut Hill, MA 02467
(617) 991-0102
(866) 509-0732 (toll-free)
http://www.mbmi.org
Superb collection of instructional tapes
and CDs

ENVIRONMENTAL AND NUTRITIONAL
CONTAMINANTS

The Environmental Working Group
1436 U Street NW, Suite 100
Washington, DC 20009
(202) 667-6982
http://www.ewg.org
Provides up-to-date information on mercury in fish, and pesticides on produce

Mercury Testing
  Sierra Club
  85 Second St., 2nd Floor
  San Francisco, CA 94105
  (415) 977-5500
  www.sierraclub.com/mercury

Omega-3 Supplement Independent Quality Assurance

International Fish Oil Standards
  Nutrasource Diagnostics
  Granbry Building, Suite 4
  130 Research Lane
  University of Guelph Research Park
  Guelph, Ontario, Canada N1G 5G3
  (877) 557-7722 (toll-free)
  www.nutrasource.ca
  Provides independent testing of omega-3
  fish oil supplements

Small Intestinal Bacterial Overgrowth and Intestinal Lactate Testing

Integrative Care Centre of Toronto
  3600 Ellesmere Road, Unit 4
  Toronto, ON M1C 4Y8
  www.thedoctors.ca

Nutritional Supplements

Genuine Health Inc.
  317 Adelaide St West, 501
  Toronto, ON M5V 1P9
  (416) 977-8765
  (877) 500-7888 (toll-free)
  www.genuinehealth.com
  For greens+ and the concentrated omega-3
  EPA called o3mega+ joy™, for the healthy
  meal replacement nutrilean+, which meets
  government guidelines, and many other
  high-quality nutritional products. Genuine
  Health is a science-based company, and
  product development is based primarily on
  filling in the nutritional voids in North
  America. They work closely with university-based scientists and have conducted
  original research on products at the
  University of Toronto.

Juvenon Inc.
  21-C Orinda Way #132
  Orinda, CA 94563-2510
  (800) 588-3666
  www.juvenon.com

ZenBev™
  Biosential Inc.
  1543 Bayview Avenue, Suite 346
  Toronto, ON M4G 3B5
  Canada
  (800) 735-4538 (toll-free)
  (416) 421-7445
  www.zenbev.com

Life Extension Foundation
  110 West Commercial Blvd.
  Ft. Lauderdale, FL 33309
  (800) 678-8989 (toll-free)
  www.lef.org

Probiotics

Lactobacillus plantarum 299V (Probiotic
  Solutions)
  Advanced BioSolutions
  ℅ Healthy Directions, LLC
  Customer Service Center
  P.O. Box 52
  Arden, NC 28704-9807
  (888) 887-7498 (toll-free)
  www.drsinatra.com

Yakult International (USA)
  3510 Torrance Blvd., Suite 216
  Torrance, CA 90503
  (310) 792-1422
  Contact: Hisashi Satoi
  e-mail hsatoi@yakultusa.com
  www.yakult.co.jp/english/

Lactobacillus GG
  Culturelle™
  ConAgra Foods
  One ConAgra Drive
  Omaha, NE 68102
  (402) 595-4000
  (888) 828-4242 (toll-free)
  e-mail: culturelle@conagrafoods.com

Align™ (*Bifidobacterium infantis* 35624)
  1 Procter & Gamble Plaza
  Cincinnati, OH 45202
  (800) 208-0112 (toll-free)
  www.aligngi.com
  Highly researched probiotic proven to
  lower inflammatory markers outside the
  gut. High-quality research shows benefit
  in irritable bowel syndrome. Beautifully
  packaged—hopefully they will remove the
  unnecessary blue food dye so that sensitive children and adults with ADHD,
  autism, chronic fatigue syndrome, and
  fibromyalgia can take advantage of this
  special strain.

Actimel by Dannon
    Dannon Consumer Response Center
    P.O. Box 90296
    Allentown, PA 18109-0296
    (877) 326-6668 (toll-free)
    www.actimel.com

BIOFEEDBACK/SUPPLIES FOR MEDITATION AND MIND-BODY EXERCISES

Biodot of Indiana Inc.
    P.O. Box 2246
    Indianapolis, IN 46206
    (800) 367-1604 (toll-free)
    http://www.stressstop.com

StressEraser
    Helicor, Inc.
    156 5th Avenue, Suite 1218
    New York, NY 10010
    www.stresseraser.com

SAUNA

SaunaRay Infrared Saunas
    (877) 992-1100 (toll-free)
    www.saunaray.com
    e-mail: info@saunaray.com

Negative Air Ion Generator
    SphereOne, Inc.
    945 Main St./P.O. Box 1013
    Silver Plum, CO 80476
    (800) 858-3229 (toll-free)
    www.sphereone.com

Cobblestone Walkway Mats
    Oregon Research Institute
    1715 Franklin Blvd.
    Eugene, OR 97403
    (541) 484-2123
    Fax: (541) 484-1108
    www.ori.org

FOOD AND BRAIN RESEARCH UPDATES

Food and Behaviour Research
    FAB Research
    Box 6066
    Nairn, Scotland
    IV12 4YN
    Telephone: 0870 756 5960
    www.fabresearch.org
    email: info@fabresearch.org
    Directors are Dr. Alex Richardson and
    Marion Ross; Food and Behaviour Research
    (FAB Research) is a charitable organiza-
    tion dedicated both to advancing scien-
    tific research into the links between
    nutrition and human behavior and to
    making the findings from such research
    available to the widest possible audience.

LACTOSE INTOLERANCE

Tony's Lactose Free Cookbook
    Drs. Anthony Campbell and Stephanie
    Matthews
    www.welstonpress.com
    Windsor Bookshop
    9a Windsor Road, Penarth
    CF64 1JB
    United Kingdom
    +44 (0)29 2070 6455
    Fax: +44 (0)29 2070 6177

BROCCOSPROUTS AND DETOX SUPPORT

Brassica Protection Products LLC,
    2400 Boston Street Suite 358
    Baltimore, Maryland 21224
    (877) 747-1277 (877-SGS-1BPP; toll-free)
    (410) 732-1200
    Fax: (410) 732-1980
    www.brassica.com
    email: mail@brassica.com

Genuine Health Inc.
    For greens+ daily detox (see above)

HEALTH FOOD CHAINS

Whole Foods Market Inc.
    550 Bowie Street
    Austin, TX 78703-4677
    (512) 477-4455
    voicemail: (512) 477-5566
    fax: (512) 482-7000
    www.wholefoodsmarket.com

Wild Oats Markets Inc.
   3375 Mitchell Lane
   Boulder, CO 80301
   (800) 494-9453 (toll-free)
   www.wildoats.com

JAPANESE FOODS

Mitsuwa Marketplace
   595 River Road
   Edgewater, NJ 07020
   (201) 941-9113
   Nine retail markets in the United States

Nippan Daido
   522 Mamaroneck Ave.
   White Plains, NY 10605
   (914) 683-6735
   Three retail markets in the United States

Online Source of Japanese Matcha, Green Tea
   Noodles, Sesame, and Polyphenol-Rich
   Chocolate: www.kenkonutrition.com

NUTRITION INFORMATION AND TRADITIONAL
REGIONAL DIETS

Oldways Preservation & Exchange Trust
   266 Beacon Street
   Boston, MA 02116
   (617) 421-5500
   www.oldwayspt.org
   Oldways is the widely respected nonprofit
   "food issues think tank" praised for trans-
   lating the complex details of nutrition science into "the familiar language of food."
   This synthesis converts high-level science
   into a consumer-friendly health-
   promotion tool for all. Jointly with the
   Harvard School of Public Health and other
   institutions, Oldways has published the
   "healthy eating pyramids," a set of unique
   dietary guides based on worldwide dietary
   traditions closely associated with good
   health.

FROZEN SEAFOOD BURGERS—SHRIMP, TUNA,
MAHI-MAHI AND SALMON

Omega Foods Ltd.
   P.O. Box 21256
   Eugene, OR 97402
   (541) 349-0731
   www.omegafoods.com

ORGANIC SOUP STOCKS WITH NO ADDED
CHEMICALS

Imagine Foods
   The Hain Celestial Group
   4600 Sleepytime Dr.
   Boulder, CO 80301
   (800) 434-4246 (toll-free)
   www.imaginefoods.com

HEALTHY SNACKS AND SALAD DRESSING/
DIPPING SAUCES WITH NO ADDED CHEMICALS

Sahale Snacks
   P.O. Box 9345
   Seattle, WA 98109
   www.sahalesnacks.com

Mrs. May's Naturals
   12436 Bell Ranch Dr.
   Santa Fe Springs, CA 90670
   (562) 906-0345
   www.mrsmays.com

The Ginger People
   Royal Pacific Foods
   Monterey, CA 93940
   (800) 551-5284 (toll-free)
   www.gingerpeople.com

ANTIOXIDANT FOODS

International Tree Nut Council
   2413 Anza Ave.
   Davis, CA 95616
   (530) 297-5895
   www.nuthealth.org

Acai Amazon Palmberry
   SAMBAZON
   927 Calle Negocio, Suite J
   San Clemente, CA 92673
   (877) SAMBAZON (toll-free)
   www.sambazon.com

Wild Blueberry Association of North America
   P.O. Box 1130
   Kennebunkport, ME 04046
   (207) 967-5024
   www.wildblueberries.com

Pomegranate Juice
   POM Wonderful, LLC
   11444 West Olympic Blvd.
   Los Angeles, CA 90064
   (310) 966-5800
   www.pomwonderful.com

About the Author

Alan C. Logan is a faculty member of Harvard Medical School's Mind-Body Institute. He graduated magna cum laude from the State University of New York and was the valedictorian upon graduation from the Canadian College of Naturopathic Medicine in 2001. The nutrition editor of the *International Journal of Naturopathic Medicine* and a regular contributor to health magazines, Alan has been published in mainstream journals such as *Nutrition, Arthritis and Rheumatology, American Journal of Hypertension, Medical Hypotheses, Hospital Physician,* and *Medical Clinics of North America.* He resides in Westchester County, New York.